Welcome to the ***"Cookbook For Diabetics and High Cholesterol: 115+ Wholesome Recipes for Diabetics and Lowering Cholesterol."*** *This cookbook is a comprehensive guide designed to support individuals managing diabetes and striving to lower their cholesterol levels through delicious and nutritious cooking.*

Living with diabetes and high cholesterol can present challenges, especially when it comes to making dietary choices that are both satisfying and beneficial to your health. This book aims to empower you with a collection of over 115 recipes that are specifically crafted to be diabetes-friendly and supportive of heart health.

Each recipe in this cookbook has been meticulously developed to ensure it meets the nutritional needs of individuals managing these health conditions, without compromising on flavor. Whether you're looking for hearty breakfast ideas, satisfying main courses, flavorful sides, or indulgent desserts, you'll find a wealth of options that cater to your dietary requirements.

Beyond just recipes, this book provides practical tips on ingredient selection, cooking techniques, and meal planning strategies that can help you navigate your culinary journey with confidence. We believe that eating well should never mean sacrificing taste, and with the recipes in this book, you'll discover how wholesome ingredients and mindful cooking can enhance both your health and your enjoyment of food.

Thank you for choosing this cookbook to support your journey towards better health. Whether you're cooking for yourself or for loved ones, we hope these recipes inspire you to create nourishing meals that nourish both body and soul.

Here's to delicious, wholesome cooking and a healthier you!

1. Grilled salmon with lemon and herbs

Ingredient:

- 4 salmon fillets (about 4•6 oz each)
- 2 tbsp olive oil
- 2 tbsp fresh lemon juice
- 1 tsp dried oregano
- 1 tsp dried basil
- 1/2 tsp garlic powder
- 1/4 tsp salt
- 1/4 tsp black pepper

Instructions:

1. Preheat grill to medium•high heat.

2. In a small bowl, whisk together the olive oil, lemon juice, oregano, basil, garlic powder, salt, and pepper.

3. Place the salmon fillets on a large plate or baking sheet. Brush the salmon evenly with the lemon•herb mixture, making sure to coat all sides.

4. Grill the salmon for 8•12 minutes, flipping halfway through, until the fish flakes easily with a fork and is cooked through.

5. Serve the grilled salmon immediately, garnished with extra lemon wedges if desired.

This recipe is diabetes•friendly and heart•healthy, as it is low in carbs, high in protein, and uses healthy fats from the salmon and olive oil. The lemon and herbs add flavor without the need for high•sodium sauces or marinades. Enjoy this delicious and nutritious grilled salmon!

2. Baked chicken with roasted vegetables

Ingredient:

- 4 boneless, skinless chicken breasts
- 2 cups mixed vegetables (such as broccoli, cauliflower, bell peppers, zucchini, onions), chopped into 1•inch pieces
- 2 tbsp olive oil
- 1 tsp dried thyme
- 1 tsp dried rosemary
- 1/2 tsp garlic powder
- 1/4 tsp salt
- 1/4 tsp black pepper

Instructions:

1. Preheat the oven to 400°F (200°C).

2. In a large baking dish or sheet pan, toss the chopped vegetables with 1 tbsp of the olive oil, 1/2 tsp of the thyme, 1/2 tsp of the rosemary, and a pinch of salt and pepper. Spread the vegetables in a single layer.

3. Place the chicken breasts on top of the vegetables. Brush the chicken with the remaining 1 tbsp of olive oil and sprinkle with the remaining 1/2 tsp each of thyme and rosemary, as well as the garlic powder, salt, and pepper.

4. Bake for 25•30 minutes, or until the chicken is cooked through (internal temperature reaches 165°F/75°C) and the vegetables are tender.

5. Serve the baked chicken and roasted vegetables immediately.

This dish is a great option for those with diabetes or high cholesterol as it is high in protein, low in carbs, and uses healthy fats from the olive oil. The roasted vegetables provide fiber, vitamins, and minerals. Adjust the cooking time as needed based on the thickness of your chicken breasts.

3. Quinoa salad with roasted vegetables

Ingredient:

- 1 cup uncooked quinoa, rinsed
- 2 cups low•sodium vegetable or chicken broth
- 1 cup chopped bell peppers (mix of red, yellow, and/or orange)
- 1 cup chopped zucchini
- 1 cup chopped red onion
- 2 tbsp olive oil
- 1 tsp dried oregano
- 1/2 tsp garlic powder
- 1/4 tsp salt
- 1/4 tsp black pepper
- 2 tbsp chopped fresh parsley
- 2 tbsp lemon juice

Instructions:

1. Preheat the oven to 400°F (200°C).

2. In a medium saucepan, combine the quinoa and broth. Bring to a boil, then reduce heat to low, cover, and simmer for 15•20 minutes, until the quinoa is cooked and the liquid is absorbed. Fluff with a fork and set aside to cool.

3. On a large baking sheet, toss the chopped bell peppers, zucchini, and red onion with the olive oil, oregano, garlic powder, salt, and pepper. Roast for 20•25 minutes, stirring halfway, until the vegetables are tender and lightly browned.

4. In a large bowl, combine the cooked quinoa, roasted vegetables, parsley, and lemon juice. Toss gently to mix.

5. Serve the quinoa salad warm or chilled.

This quinoa salad is a great option for those with diabetes or high cholesterol as it is high in fiber, protein, and healthy fats, while being low in carbs and sodium. The roasted vegetables add flavor and nutrients. Adjust the amounts of vegetables to your liking.

4. Lentil soup with spinach

Ingredient:

- 1 cup dry brown or green lentils, rinsed
- 4 cups low•sodium vegetable or chicken broth
- 1 tbsp olive oil
- 1 onion, diced
- 2 carrots, peeled and diced
- 2 celery stalks, diced
- 3 garlic cloves, minced
- 1 tsp ground cumin
- 1 tsp dried oregano
- 1/4 tsp red pepper flakes (optional)
- 1/4 tsp salt
- 1/4 tsp black pepper
- 4 cups fresh spinach, chopped
- 2 tbsp lemon juice

Instructions:

1. In a large pot, combine the lentils and broth. Bring to a boil, then reduce heat and simmer for 15•20 minutes, until the lentils are tender.

2. In a separate skillet, heat the olive oil over medium heat. Add the onion, carrots, and celery, and sauté for 5•7 minutes, until the vegetables are softened.

3. Add the garlic, cumin, oregano, and red pepper flakes (if using) to the skillet. Cook for 1 minute, until fragrant.

4. Transfer the sautéed vegetables to the pot with the cooked lentils. Stir in the salt and pepper.

5. Add the chopped spinach to the soup and cook for 2•3 minutes, until the spinach is wilted.

6. Remove the soup from heat and stir in the lemon juice.

7. Serve the lentil soup hot, garnished with additional lemon wedges if desired.

This lentil soup is a great option for those with diabetes or high cholesterol as it is high in fiber, protein, and nutrients, while being low in carbs and sodium. The spinach adds additional vitamins and minerals.

5. Turkey chili with beans

Ingredient:

- 1 lb ground turkey
- 1 tbsp olive oil
- 1 onion, diced
- 3 garlic cloves, minced
- 2 tbsp chili powder
- 1 tsp ground cumin
- 1 tsp dried oregano
- 1/4 tsp cayenne pepper (optional)
- 1 (15 oz) can no•salt•added diced tomatoes
- 1 (15 oz) can no•salt•added kidney beans, rinsed and drained
- 1 (15 oz) can no•salt•added black beans, rinsed and drained
- 1 cup low•sodium chicken or vegetable broth
- 1/4 tsp salt
- 1/4 tsp black pepper
- 2 tbsp chopped fresh cilantro (for garnish)

Instructions:

1. In a large pot or Dutch oven, heat the olive oil over medium•high heat. Add the ground turkey and cook, breaking it up with a wooden spoon, until browned, about 5•7 minutes.

2. Add the diced onion and minced garlic to the pot. Cook for 2•3 minutes, until the onion is translucent.

3. Stir in the chili powder, cumin, oregano, and cayenne (if using). Cook for 1 minute to toast the spices.

4. Add the diced tomatoes, kidney beans, black beans, and broth. Bring the mixture to a simmer.

5. Reduce the heat to medium•low and let the chili simmer for 20•25 minutes, stirring occasionally, until the flavors have melded and the chili has thickened.

6. Season with salt and black pepper. Serve the turkey chili hot, garnished with chopped fresh cilantro.

This turkey chili is a great option for those with diabetes or high cholesterol as it is high in protein, fiber, and nutrients, while being low in carbs and sodium. The beans provide complex carbs and additional fiber. Adjust the amount of cayenne pepper to your desired level of spice.

6. Stir•fried tofu with broccoli

Ingredient:

- 1 block (14 oz) extra•firm tofu, drained and cubed
- 2 tbsp low•sodium soy sauce or tamari
- 1 tbsp rice vinegar
- 1 tsp sesame oil
- 1 tbsp cornstarch
- 2 tbsp olive oil
- 3 cups broccoli florets
- 2 garlic cloves, minced
- 1 tsp grated fresh ginger
- 1/4 tsp red pepper flakes (optional)
- 2 tbsp chopped green onions (for garnish)

Instructions:

1. In a medium bowl, combine the cubed tofu, soy sauce, rice vinegar, sesame oil, and cornstarch. Toss gently to coat the tofu.

2. In a large skillet or wok, heat the olive oil over medium•high heat. Add the broccoli florets and stir•fry for 3•4 minutes, until the broccoli is crisp•tender.

3. Add the garlic, ginger, and red pepper flakes (if using) to the skillet. Cook for 1 minute, until fragrant.

4. Add the marinated tofu to the skillet and continue to stir•fry for 5•7 minutes, until the tofu is lightly browned and the sauce has thickened.

5. Remove the skillet from heat and garnish the stir•fried tofu and broccoli with the chopped green onions.

6. Serve immediately, over steamed brown rice or quinoa if desired.

This stir•fried tofu and broccoli dish is a great option for those with diabetes or high cholesterol. It's high in protein from the tofu, low in carbs, and uses healthy fats from the olive oil. The broccoli provides fiber, vitamins, and minerals. Adjust the amount of red pepper flakes to your desired level of spice.

7. Zucchini noodles with marinara sauce

Ingredient:

- 4 medium zucchini, spiralized or julienned into noodles
- 1 tbsp olive oil
- 3 garlic cloves, minced
- 1 (28 oz) can no•salt•added diced tomatoes
- 2 tbsp tomato paste
- 1 tsp dried oregano
- 1/4 tsp red pepper flakes (optional)
- 1/4 tsp salt
- 1/4 tsp black pepper
- 2 tbsp chopped fresh basil

Instructions:

1. In a large skillet, heat the olive oil over medium heat. Add the minced garlic and cook for 1 minute, until fragrant.

2. Add the diced tomatoes, tomato paste, oregano, red pepper flakes (if using), salt, and pepper. Stir to combine.

3. Bring the sauce to a simmer and let it cook for 10•15 minutes, stirring occasionally, until the sauce has thickened slightly.

4. Add the spiralized or julienned zucchini noodles to the sauce and toss to coat. Cook for 2•3 minutes, just until the zucchini noodles are tender but still have a bit of bite.

5. Remove the skillet from heat and stir in the chopped fresh basil.

6. Serve the zucchini noodles with the marinara sauce immediately.

This dish is a great option for those with diabetes or high cholesterol as it is low in carbs, high in fiber, and uses healthy fats from the olive oil. The zucchini noodles provide a nutritious, low•calorie alternative to traditional pasta, and the marinara sauce is packed with antioxidants from the tomatoes.

8. Cauliflower rice stir•fry

Ingredient:

- 1 head of cauliflower, riced (about 4 cups riced cauliflower)
- 2 tbsp olive oil
- 1 onion, diced
- 2 garlic cloves, minced
- 1 cup sliced mushrooms
- 1 cup chopped broccoli florets
- 1 red bell pepper, diced
- 2 tbsp low•sodium soy sauce or tamari
- 1 tsp sesame oil
- 1/4 tsp ground ginger
- 1/4 tsp red pepper flakes (optional)
- 2 tbsp chopped fresh cilantro (for garnish)

Instructions:

1. In a food processor, pulse the cauliflower florets until they are broken down into small, rice•like pieces. Set aside.

2. In a large skillet or wok, heat the olive oil over medium•high heat. Add the diced onion and sauté for 2•3 minutes, until translucent.

3. Add the minced garlic, sliced mushrooms, chopped broccoli, and diced red bell pepper. Stir•fry for 4•5 minutes, until the vegetables are tender•crisp.

4. Add the riced cauliflower to the skillet. Pour in the soy sauce, sesame oil, ground ginger, and red pepper flakes (if using). Stir to combine.

5. Continue to stir•fry the cauliflower rice mixture for 3•4 minutes, until the cauliflower is tender but still has a bit of bite.

6. Remove the skillet from heat and stir in the chopped fresh cilantro.

7. Serve the cauliflower rice stir•fry immediately.

This cauliflower rice stir•fry is a great option for those with diabetes or high cholesterol. It's low in carbs, high in fiber, and uses healthy fats from the olive oil. The vegetables provide a variety of vitamins, minerals, and antioxidants.

9. Greek salad with feta cheese

Ingredient:

- 6 cups chopped romaine lettuce
- 1 cup cherry tomatoes, halved
- 1 cucumber, diced
- 1/2 red onion, thinly sliced
- 1/2 cup pitted kalamata olives, halved
- 1/2 cup crumbled feta cheese
- 2 tbsp olive oil
- 1 tbsp red wine vinegar
- 1 tsp dried oregano
- 1/4 tsp salt
- 1/4 tsp black pepper

Instructions:

1. In a large salad bowl, combine the chopped romaine lettuce, cherry tomatoes, diced cucumber, sliced red onion, and halved kalamata olives.

2. Sprinkle the crumbled feta cheese over the top of the salad.

3. In a small bowl, whisk together the olive oil, red wine vinegar, dried oregano, salt, and black pepper to make the dressing.

4. Drizzle the dressing over the salad and toss gently to coat.

5. Serve the Greek salad immediately.

This Greek salad is a great option for those with diabetes or high cholesterol. It's high in fiber, vitamins, and healthy fats from the olive oil and feta cheese, while being low in carbs. The vegetables provide antioxidants, and the olives and feta add a flavorful Mediterranean twist.

Remember to watch your portion sizes, as the feta cheese and olives can be higher in sodium. You can also adjust the amount of feta cheese to your liking.

10. Baked cod with tomatoes and olives

Ingredient:

- 4 cod fillets (about 4•6 oz each)
- 1 (14.5 oz) can diced tomatoes, no salt added
- 1/2 cup pitted kalamata olives, halved
- 2 tbsp olive oil
- 2 garlic cloves, minced
- 1 tsp dried oregano
- 1/4 tsp salt
- 1/4 tsp black pepper
- 2 tbsp chopped fresh parsley

Instructions:

1. Preheat the oven to 400°F (200°C).

2. In a baking dish or oven•safe skillet, combine the diced tomatoes, olives, olive oil, garlic, oregano, salt, and pepper. Stir to mix well.

3. Place the cod fillets on top of the tomato•olive mixture, making sure the fish is evenly spaced.

4. Bake for 15•20 minutes, or until the cod is cooked through and flakes easily with a fork.

5. Remove the dish from the oven and sprinkle the chopped parsley over the top.

6. Serve the baked cod immediately, spooning the tomato•olive mixture over the fish.

This baked cod dish is a great option for those with diabetes or high cholesterol as it is high in protein, low in carbs, and uses healthy fats from the olive oil. The tomatoes and olives provide antioxidants and healthy fats, while the parsley adds fresh flavor.

11. Shrimp and vegetable skewers

Ingredient:

- 1 lb large shrimp, peeled and deveined
- 1 red bell pepper, cut into 1•inch pieces
- 1 zucchini, cut into 1•inch pieces
- 1 red onion, cut into 1•inch pieces
- 8 cherry tomatoes
- 2 tbsp olive oil
- 1 tbsp lemon juice
- 1 tsp dried oregano
- 1/4 tsp salt
- 1/4 tsp black pepper

Instructions:

1. Preheat your grill or grill pan to medium•high heat.

2. In a large bowl, combine the shrimp, bell pepper, zucchini, red onion, and cherry tomatoes.

3. In a small bowl, whisk together the olive oil, lemon juice, oregano, salt, and black pepper.

4. Pour the marinade over the shrimp and vegetables and toss to coat everything evenly.

5. Thread the shrimp and vegetables onto skewers, alternating the ingredients.

6. Grill the skewers for 8•10 minutes, turning occasionally, until the shrimp are opaque and the vegetables are tender.

7. Serve the grilled shrimp and vegetable skewers immediately.

This dish is a great option for those with diabetes or high cholesterol as it is high in protein from the shrimp, low in carbs, and uses healthy fats from the olive oil. The variety of vegetables provides fiber, vitamins, and minerals.

You can adjust the types of vegetables used based on your preferences. Serve the skewers with a side of roasted sweet potatoes or a fresh salad for a complete, balanced meal.

12. Eggplant parmesan

Ingredient:

- 1 large eggplant, sliced into 1/2•inch thick rounds
- 1 cup whole wheat breadcrumbs
- 1/2 cup grated Parmesan cheese
- 1 tsp dried oregano
- 1/2 tsp garlic powder
- 1/4 tsp salt
- 1/4 tsp black pepper
- 1 egg, beaten
- 1 (24 oz) jar no•sugar•added marinara sauce
- 1 cup shredded part•skim mozzarella cheese

Instructions:

1. Preheat the oven to 375°F (190°C). Line a baking sheet with parchment paper.

2. In a shallow bowl, combine the breadcrumbs, Parmesan, oregano, garlic powder, salt, and pepper.

3. Dip the eggplant slices into the beaten egg, then coat them in the breadcrumb mixture, pressing gently to adhere.

4. Arrange the breaded eggplant slices in a single layer on the prepared baking sheet.

5. Bake for 20•25 minutes, flipping the slices halfway, until the eggplant is tender and the breading is golden brown.

6. Spread a thin layer of marinara sauce in the bottom of a 9x13•inch baking dish. Arrange the baked eggplant slices in a single layer on top of the sauce.

7. Top the eggplant with the remaining marinara sauce and the shredded mozzarella cheese.

8. Bake for an additional 15•20 minutes, until the cheese is melted and bubbly. Let the eggplant parmesan cool for 5 minutes before serving.

This baked eggplant parmesan is a healthier alternative to the traditional fried version. It's lower in carbs, uses whole wheat breadcrumbs, and features part•skim mozzarella cheese, making it a better choice for those with diabetes or high cholesterol. Enjoy this dish as part of a balanced, nutrient•dense meal.

13. Spinach and mushroom frittata

Ingredient:

- 8 large eggs
- 1/4 cup unsweetened almond milk (or low•fat milk)
- 1/4 tsp salt
- 1/4 tsp black pepper
- 1 tbsp olive oil
- 8 oz sliced mushrooms
- 2 cups fresh spinach, chopped
- 1/4 cup shredded low•fat cheddar cheese

Instructions:

1. Preheat your oven to 375°F (190°C).

2. In a medium bowl, whisk together the eggs, almond milk, salt, and black pepper. Set aside.

3. In a 9•inch oven•safe non•stick skillet, heat the olive oil over medium heat. Add the sliced mushrooms and sauté for 5•7 minutes, until they are tender and lightly browned.

4. Add the chopped spinach to the skillet and cook for 2•3 minutes, until the spinach is wilted.

5. Pour the egg mixture over the mushrooms and spinach. Sprinkle the shredded cheddar cheese evenly over the top.

6. Transfer the skillet to the preheated oven and bake for 18•22 minutes, or until the frittata is set and the cheese is melted.

7. Remove the frittata from the oven and let it cool for 5 minutes before slicing and serving.

This spinach and mushroom frittata is a great option for those with diabetes or high cholesterol. It's high in protein, low in carbs, and uses healthy fats from the olive oil and low•fat cheese. The spinach and mushrooms provide fiber, vitamins, and minerals.

You can serve the frittata with a side of roasted vegetables or a fresh salad for a complete, balanced meal.

14. Chickpea curry with brown rice

Ingredient:

- 1 cup uncooked brown rice
- 2 tbsp olive oil
- 1 onion, diced
- 3 garlic cloves, minced
- 1 tbsp grated fresh ginger
- 2 tsp garam masala
- 1 tsp ground cumin
- 1/2 tsp ground coriander
- 1/4 tsp cayenne pepper (optional)
- 1 (15 oz) can chickpeas, rinsed and drained
- 1 (14.5 oz) can diced tomatoes, no salt added
- 1 cup low•sodium vegetable or chicken broth
- 1/2 cup full•fat coconut milk
- 1/4 tsp salt
- 1/4 tsp black pepper
- 2 cups baby spinach, chopped
- 2 tbsp chopped fresh cilantro

Instructions:

1. Cook the brown rice according to package instructions.

2. In a large skillet or saucepan, heat the olive oil over medium heat. Add the onion and sauté for 5•7 minutes, until translucent.

3. Add the garlic and ginger, and cook for 1 minute, until fragrant.

4. Stir in the garam masala, cumin, coriander, and cayenne (if using). Cook for 1 minute.

5. Add the chickpeas, diced tomatoes, broth, and coconut milk. Bring to a simmer and cook for 10•15 minutes, until the sauce has thickened slightly.

6. Season with salt and pepper. Stir in the chopped spinach and cook for 2•3 minutes, until the spinach is wilted. Serve the chickpea curry over the cooked brown rice, garnished with fresh cilantro.

This chickpea curry is a great option for those with diabetes or high cholesterol as it is high in fiber, protein, and healthy fats, while being low in carbs and sodium. The brown rice provides complex carbs, and the spinach adds additional nutrients.

15. Turkey and vegetable stir•fry

Ingredient:

• 1 lb ground turkey
• 2 tbsp low•sodium soy sauce or tamari
• 1 tbsp rice vinegar
• 1 tsp sesame oil
• 2 tbsp olive oil
• 1 onion, sliced
• 2 cups broccoli florets
• 1 red bell pepper, sliced
• 2 cups sliced mushrooms
• 3 garlic cloves, minced
• 1 tbsp grated fresh ginger
• 1/4 tsp red pepper flakes (optional)
• 2 cups cooked brown rice, for serving

Instructions:

1. In a medium bowl, combine the ground turkey, soy sauce, rice vinegar, and sesame oil. Mix well and set aside.

2. In a large skillet or wok, heat the olive oil over medium•high heat.

3. Add the sliced onion and stir•fry for 2•3 minutes, until translucent.

4. Add the broccoli florets, sliced red bell pepper, and sliced mushrooms. Stir•fry for 4•5 minutes, until the vegetables are tender•crisp.

5. Push the vegetables to the side of the skillet and add the marinated ground turkey. Cook the turkey, breaking it up with a wooden spoon, for 5•7 minutes, until no longer pink.

6. Add the minced garlic, grated ginger, and red pepper flakes (if using). Stir everything together and cook for 1 minute, until fragrant. Serve the turkey and vegetable stir•fry over the cooked brown rice.

This turkey and vegetable stir•fry is a great option for those with diabetes or high cholesterol. It's high in protein, low in carbs, and uses healthy fats from the olive oil. The variety of vegetables provides fiber, vitamins, and minerals.

You can adjust the types of vegetables used based on your preferences. Serve this dish with a side of steamed greens for a complete, balanced meal.

16. Baked sweet potato with black beans

Ingredient:

- 4 medium sweet potatoes
- 1 (15 oz) can no•salt•added black beans, rinsed and drained
- 1 tbsp olive oil
- 1 tsp ground cumin
- 1/2 tsp chili powder
- 1/4 tsp garlic powder
- 1/4 tsp salt
- 1/4 tsp black pepper
- 2 tbsp chopped fresh cilantro (for garnish)

Instructions:

1. Preheat your oven to 400°F (200°C).

2. Wash the sweet potatoes and prick them several times with a fork. Place the sweet potatoes directly on the oven rack and bake for 45•60 minutes, until they are tender when pierced with a fork.

3. In a medium bowl, combine the rinsed and drained black beans, olive oil, cumin, chili powder, garlic powder, salt, and black pepper. Stir to coat the beans evenly.

4. Once the sweet potatoes are cooked, remove them from the oven and let them cool for 5 minutes.

5. Slice each sweet potato in half lengthwise and top with the seasoned black bean mixture.

6. Garnish the baked sweet potatoes with the chopped fresh cilantro.

7. Serve the sweet potatoes with black beans immediately.

This dish is a great option for those with diabetes or high cholesterol. The sweet potatoes are high in fiber, vitamins, and complex carbs, while the black beans provide protein and additional fiber. The olive oil and spices add flavor without the need for high•sodium sauces or toppings.

Adjust the amount of chili powder to your desired level of spice. Enjoy this nutritious and satisfying meal.

17. Grilled chicken Caesar salad

Ingredient:

- 4 boneless, skinless chicken breasts
- 1 tbsp olive oil
- 1/2 tsp garlic powder
- 1/4 tsp salt
- 1/4 tsp black pepper
- 6 cups chopped romaine lettuce
- 1/2 cup shredded Parmesan cheese
- 2 tbsp low•fat Caesar dressing
- 2 tbsp whole wheat croutons (optional)

Instructions:

1. Preheat your grill or grill pan to medium•high heat.

2. Brush the chicken breasts with the olive oil and season them with the garlic powder, salt, and black pepper.

3. Grill the chicken for 6•8 minutes per side, or until it's cooked through and reaches an internal temperature of 165°F (75°C).

4. Remove the chicken from the grill and let it rest for 5 minutes before slicing it into strips.

5. In a large salad bowl, combine the chopped romaine lettuce, sliced grilled chicken, shredded Parmesan cheese, and Caesar dressing. Toss gently to coat.

6. If desired, top the salad with the whole wheat croutons.

7. Serve the grilled chicken Caesar salad immediately.

This grilled chicken Caesar salad is a great option for those with diabetes or high cholesterol. It's high in protein from the grilled chicken, low in carbs, and uses a low•fat Caesar dressing. The romaine lettuce provides fiber and nutrients, while the Parmesan cheese adds flavor without too much saturated fat.

You can adjust the amount of dressing used to your preference, and the croutons are optional if you want to further reduce the carb content.

18. Tuna salad with avocado

Ingredient:

- 2 (5 oz) cans of water•packed tuna, drained
- 1 ripe avocado, diced
- 2 tbsp plain Greek yogurt
- 1 tbsp lemon juice
- 1 tbsp chopped fresh parsley
- 1/4 tsp salt
- 1/4 tsp black pepper
- 2 cups mixed greens

Instructions:

1. In a medium bowl, gently mix together the drained tuna, diced avocado, Greek yogurt, lemon juice, chopped parsley, salt, and black pepper until well combined.

2. Serve the tuna salad on a bed of mixed greens.

Optional Serving Suggestions:
- Scoop the tuna salad into halved avocado shells
- Serve the tuna salad on whole grain crackers or toast
- Add diced celery or red onion for extra crunch and flavor

This tuna salad with avocado is a great option for those with diabetes or high cholesterol. It's high in protein from the tuna, healthy fats from the avocado, and low in carbs. The Greek yogurt provides creaminess without the need for mayonnaise.

The mixed greens add fiber, vitamins, and minerals to the dish. You can adjust the amount of lemon juice, parsley, salt, and pepper to suit your taste preferences.

This tuna salad makes a satisfying and nutritious lunch or light dinner. Enjoy it on its own or with your choice of healthy accompaniments.

19. Roasted Brussels sprouts with bacon

Ingredient:

- 1 lb Brussels sprouts, trimmed and halved
- 2 tbsp olive oil
- 1/4 tsp salt
- 1/4 tsp black pepper
- 4 slices of bacon, cooked and crumbled

Instructions:

1. Preheat the oven to 400°F (200°C).

2. In a large bowl, toss the Brussels sprouts with the olive oil, salt, and pepper until the sprouts are evenly coated.

3. Spread the Brussels sprouts in a single layer on a baking sheet.

4. Roast for 20•25 minutes, tossing halfway, until the Brussels sprouts are tender and lightly browned.

5. Remove the roasted Brussels sprouts from the oven and sprinkle the crumbled bacon over the top.

6. Serve the roasted Brussels sprouts with bacon immediately.

This recipe is a good option for those with diabetes or high cholesterol, as long as portion sizes are kept in check. The Brussels sprouts are a nutrient•dense vegetable, and the bacon provides a small amount of flavor without overwhelming the dish. Be mindful of the sodium content from the bacon, and consider using a lower•sodium variety if available.

Remember to enjoy this dish in moderation as part of a balanced, healthy diet. The key is to focus on the nutritious Brussels sprouts and use the bacon as a garnish rather than the main component.

20. Baked tilapia with asparagus

Ingredient:

- 4 tilapia fillets (about 4•6 oz each)
- 1 lb asparagus, trimmed
- 2 tbsp olive oil, divided
- 1 tsp lemon zest
- 2 tbsp lemon juice
- 1 tsp dried dill
- 1/4 tsp salt
- 1/4 tsp black pepper

Instructions:

1. Preheat your oven to 400°F (200°C).

2. In a large baking dish or sheet pan, toss the trimmed asparagus with 1 tbsp of the olive oil. Spread the asparagus in a single layer.

3. Place the tilapia fillets on top of the asparagus. Drizzle the remaining 1 tbsp of olive oil over the fish.

4. In a small bowl, combine the lemon zest, lemon juice, dried dill, salt, and black pepper. Drizzle this mixture over the tilapia fillets.

5. Bake for 15•20 minutes, or until the tilapia is cooked through and flakes easily with a fork, and the asparagus is tender•crisp.

6. Serve the baked tilapia and asparagus immediately.

This baked tilapia and asparagus dish is a great option for those with diabetes or high cholesterol. Tilapia is a lean, mild•flavored fish that is high in protein and low in mercury. The asparagus provides fiber, vitamins, and minerals.

The lemon, dill, and olive oil add flavor without the need for high•sodium sauces or butter. This dish is low in carbs and uses healthy fats, making it a nutritious and delicious choice.

Adjust the cooking time as needed based on the thickness of your tilapia fillets. Enjoy this easy and healthy baked fish and vegetable meal.

21. Spinach and feta stuffed chicken breast

Ingredient:

- 4 boneless, skinless chicken breasts
- 2 cups fresh spinach, chopped
- 1/2 cup crumbled feta cheese
- 2 tbsp olive oil
- 1 garlic clove, minced
- 1/4 tsp dried oregano
- 1/4 tsp salt
- 1/4 tsp black pepper

Instructions:

1. Preheat your oven to 400°F (200°C).

2. In a medium bowl, combine the chopped spinach, crumbled feta cheese, 1 tbsp of the olive oil, minced garlic, dried oregano, salt, and black pepper. Mix well.

3. Using a sharp knife, cut a pocket into the side of each chicken breast, being careful not to cut all the way through.

4. Stuff the spinach and feta mixture evenly into the pockets of the chicken breasts.

5. In a large oven•safe skillet or baking dish, heat the remaining 1 tbsp of olive oil over medium•high heat.

6. Add the stuffed chicken breasts to the skillet and sear for 2•3 minutes per side to get a nice golden•brown crust.

7. Transfer the skillet to the preheated oven and bake for 20•25 minutes, or until the chicken is cooked through and the internal temperature reaches 165°F (75°C).

8. Remove the stuffed chicken breasts from the oven and let them rest for 5 minutes before serving.

This spinach and feta stuffed chicken breast is a great option for those with diabetes or high cholesterol. It's high in protein, low in carbs, and uses healthy fats from the olive oil and feta cheese. The spinach provides fiber, vitamins, and minerals.

Serve the stuffed chicken breasts with a side of roasted vegetables or a fresh salad for a complete, balanced meal.

22. Quinoa stuffed bell peppers

Ingredient:

- 4 medium bell peppers (any color)
- 1 cup cooked quinoa
- 1 (15 oz) can no•salt•added black beans, rinsed and drained
- 1 cup diced tomatoes
- 1/2 cup crumbled feta cheese
- 2 tbsp chopped fresh cilantro
- 1 tsp ground cumin
- 1/4 tsp salt
- 1/4 tsp black pepper

Instructions:

1. Preheat your oven to 375°F (190°C).

2. Cut the bell peppers in half lengthwise and remove the seeds and membranes. Place the pepper halves in a baking dish.

3. In a medium bowl, combine the cooked quinoa, black beans, diced tomatoes, crumbled feta cheese, chopped cilantro, cumin, salt, and black pepper. Stir to mix well.

4. Spoon the quinoa mixture evenly into the bell pepper halves, packing it in gently.

5. Cover the baking dish with foil and bake for 25•30 minutes, or until the peppers are tender.

6. Remove the foil and bake for an additional 5 minutes to lightly brown the tops of the stuffed peppers.

7. Serve the quinoa stuffed bell peppers warm.

This dish is a great option for those with diabetes or high cholesterol. Quinoa is a high•protein, high•fiber grain, and the black beans provide additional fiber and protein. The feta cheese adds flavor without too much saturated fat.

The bell peppers provide vitamins, minerals, and antioxidants. This meal is well•balanced and nutrient•dense, making it a healthy choice for those with dietary restrictions.

Adjust the amount of feta cheese or spices to your personal taste preferences. Enjoy this delicious and nutritious stuffed pepper dish!

23. Lentil and vegetable stew

Ingredient:

• 1 cup dry brown or green lentils, rinsed
• 4 cups vegetable broth
• 1 tablespoon olive oil
• 1 onion, diced
• 3 cloves garlic, minced
• 2 carrots, peeled and diced
• 2 celery stalks, diced
• 1 bell pepper, diced
• 1 (14.5 oz) can diced tomatoes
• 2 teaspoons dried thyme
• 1 teaspoon dried oregano
• 1/2 teaspoon smoked paprika
• Salt and black pepper to taste
• Chopped parsley for garnish (optional)

Instructions:

1. In a large pot, combine the lentils and vegetable broth. Bring to a boil, then reduce heat and simmer for 15•20 minutes, until lentils are tender.

2. In a large skillet, heat the olive oil over medium heat. Add the onion and sauté for 5 minutes until translucent.

3. Add the garlic, carrots, celery and bell pepper. Sauté for 5•7 minutes until vegetables are starting to soften.

4. Add the sautéed vegetables, diced tomatoes, thyme, oregano and smoked paprika to the pot with the cooked lentils. Stir to combine.

5. Season with salt and pepper to taste.

6. Simmer the stew for 15•20 minutes, allowing the flavors to meld.

7. Serve hot, garnished with chopped parsley if desired. Enjoy!

This hearty lentil and vegetable stew is packed with fiber, protein and nutrients. It's a delicious and comforting meatless meal.

24. Turkey meatballs with zucchini noodles

Ingredient:

For the Turkey Meatballs:
- 1 lb ground turkey
- 1/4 cup whole wheat breadcrumbs
- 1 egg, beaten
- 2 tbsp grated Parmesan cheese
- 2 garlic cloves, minced
- 1 tsp dried oregano
- 1/4 tsp salt
- 1/4 tsp black pepper

For the Zucchini Noodles:
- 3 medium zucchini, spiralized or julienned
- 1 tbsp olive oil
- 2 cups no•sugar•added marinara sauce

Instructions:

1. Preheat your oven to 400°F (200°C). Line a baking sheet with parchment paper.

2. Make the turkey meatballs: In a medium bowl, combine the ground turkey, breadcrumbs, beaten egg, Parmesan cheese, minced garlic, dried oregano, salt, and black pepper. Mix well until the ingredients are evenly distributed.

3. Roll the turkey mixture into 1•inch meatballs and place them on the prepared baking sheet.

4. Bake the meatballs for 18•20 minutes, or until they are cooked through and no longer pink in the center.

5. While the meatballs are baking, prepare the zucchini noodles. In a large skillet, heat the olive oil over medium heat.

6. Add the spiralized or julienned zucchini noodles to the skillet and sauté for 3•5 minutes, until the noodles are tender but still have a bit of bite.

7. Remove the zucchini noodles from the heat and toss them with the no•sugar•added marinara sauce. Serve the baked turkey meatballs over the zucchini noodles.

This turkey meatball and zucchini noodle dish is a great option for those with diabetes or high cholesterol. The turkey meatballs are a lean protein, and the zucchini noodles provide a low•carb, fiber•rich alternative to traditional pasta.

The marinara sauce adds flavor without too much added sugar or sodium. This meal is well•balanced and nutritious, making it a great choice for those with dietary restrictions.

25. Baked eggplant with tomato sauce

Ingredient:

- 1 large eggplant, sliced into 1/2•inch thick rounds
- 2 tablespoons olive oil
- Salt and black pepper to taste
- 1 (28 oz) can crushed tomatoes
- 2 cloves garlic, minced
- 1 teaspoon dried oregano
- 1/4 cup grated Parmesan cheese
- 1 cup shredded mozzarella cheese

Instructions:

1. Preheat oven to 400°F. Line a baking sheet with parchment paper.

2. Arrange the eggplant slices in a single layer on the prepared baking sheet. Brush both sides of the eggplant with olive oil and season with salt and pepper.

3. Bake for 20•25 minutes, flipping halfway, until the eggplant is tender and lightly browned.

4. Meanwhile, in a medium saucepan, combine the crushed tomatoes, garlic, and oregano. Simmer for 10 minutes, stirring occasionally.

5. Spread a thin layer of the tomato sauce in the bottom of a 9x13 inch baking dish. Arrange the baked eggplant slices in a single layer on top of the sauce.

6. Top the eggplant with the remaining tomato sauce, then sprinkle with the Parmesan and mozzarella cheeses.

7. Bake for 15•20 minutes, until the cheese is melted and bubbly.

8. Let cool for 5 minutes before serving.

Serve the baked eggplant with tomato sauce warm, garnished with fresh basil or parsley if desired. This makes a delicious vegetarian main dish or side. Enjoy!

26. Grilled shrimp with mango salsa

Ingredient:

For the Mango Salsa:
- 1 ripe mango, diced
- 1/2 red onion, finely chopped
- 1 jalapeño, seeded and finely chopped
- 2 tbsp chopped fresh cilantro
- 1 tbsp lime juice
- 1/4 tsp salt

For the Grilled Shrimp:
- 1 lb large shrimp, peeled and deveined
- 1 tbsp olive oil
- 1 tsp chili powder
- 1/4 tsp salt
- 1/4 tsp black pepper

Instructions:

1. Make the mango salsa: In a medium bowl, combine the diced mango, chopped red onion, jalapeño, cilantro, lime juice, and 1/4 tsp of salt. Stir to mix well and set aside.

2. Prepare the shrimp: In a large bowl, toss the shrimp with the olive oil, chili powder, 1/4 tsp of salt, and black pepper until evenly coated.

3. Preheat your grill or grill pan to medium•high heat.

4. Grill the shrimp for 2•3 minutes per side, or until they are opaque and cooked through.

5. Serve the grilled shrimp immediately, topped with the fresh mango salsa.

This grilled shrimp with mango salsa is a great option for those with diabetes or high cholesterol. The shrimp is a lean protein, and the mango salsa provides a sweet and tangy contrast with healthy fats from the olive oil.

The mango, onion, and jalapeño in the salsa add fiber, vitamins, and antioxidants. This dish is low in carbs and uses minimal added salt, making it a nutritious and flavorful choice.

Adjust the amount of jalapeño in the salsa to your desired level of spice. Enjoy this delicious and healthy grilled shrimp dish!

27. Cauliflower crust pizza with vegetables

Ingredient:

For the Cauliflower Crust:
- 1 head of cauliflower, riced
(about 4 cups riced cauliflower)
- 1 egg, beaten
- 1/2 cup shredded part•skim mozzarella cheese
- 2 tbsp grated Parmesan cheese
- 1/4 tsp garlic powder
- 1/4 tsp dried oregano
- 1/4 tsp salt

For the Toppings:
- 1/2 cup no•sugar•added marinara sauce
- 1 cup sliced mushrooms
- 1 cup chopped bell peppers
- 1 cup baby spinach leaves
- 1/2 cup shredded part•skim mozzarella cheese

Instructions:

1. Preheat your oven to 400°F (200°C). Line a baking sheet with parchment paper.

2. Make the cauliflower crust: In a food processor, pulse the cauliflower florets until they are broken down into small, rice•like pieces. Transfer the riced cauliflower to a clean kitchen towel and squeeze out as much moisture as possible.

3. In a medium bowl, combine the riced cauliflower, beaten egg, mozzarella cheese, Parmesan cheese, garlic powder, dried oregano, and salt. Mix well.

4. Press the cauliflower mixture onto the prepared baking sheet, forming a thin, even crust.

5. Bake the cauliflower crust for 20•25 minutes, until it's golden brown and cooked through.

6. Remove the crust from the oven and top it with the marinara sauce, sliced mushrooms, chopped bell peppers, baby spinach leaves, and the remaining 1/2 cup of shredded mozzarella cheese.

7. Return the pizza to the oven and bake for an additional 10•15 minutes, or until the cheese is melted and bubbly. Slice and serve the cauliflower crust pizza immediately.

This cauliflower crust pizza is a great option for those with diabetes or high cholesterol. The cauliflower crust is low in carbs, and the vegetable toppings provide fiber, vitamins, and minerals. The cheese adds protein and healthy fats.

28. Greek yogurt parfait with berries

Ingredient:

- 2 cups plain Greek yogurt
- 1 cup fresh berries (such as blueberries, raspberries, or strawberries)
- 2 tbsp chopped walnuts or sliced almonds
- 1 tbsp honey (optional)

Instructions:

1. In a parfait glass or small bowl, layer the ingredients in the following order:
    - 1/2 cup Greek yogurt
    - 1/4 cup fresh berries
    - 1 tbsp chopped nuts
    - Repeat the layers

2. If desired, drizzle 1 tsp of honey over the top of the parfait.

3. Serve the Greek yogurt parfait immediately.

This Greek yogurt parfait is a great option for those with diabetes or high cholesterol. It's high in protein from the Greek yogurt, and the berries provide fiber, vitamins, and antioxidants.

The nuts add healthy fats and a crunchy texture. The honey is optional, as the parfait is already naturally sweet from the berries.

You can use a variety of berries, such as blueberries, raspberries, strawberries, or a mix. Adjust the amounts of each ingredient to your taste preferences.

This parfait makes a delicious and nutritious breakfast, snack, or light dessert. It's easy to prepare and can be made ahead of time for a quick and healthy option.

29. Baked chicken with artichokes

Ingredient:

- 4 boneless, skinless chicken breasts
- 1 (14 oz) can artichoke hearts, drained and quartered
- 2 tbsp olive oil
- 2 tbsp lemon juice
- 2 garlic cloves, minced
- 1 tsp dried oregano
- 1/4 tsp salt
- 1/4 tsp black pepper
- 1/4 cup grated Parmesan cheese

Instructions:

1. Preheat your oven to 400°F (200°C).

2. In a large baking dish, arrange the chicken breasts in a single layer.

3. In a medium bowl, combine the quartered artichoke hearts, olive oil, lemon juice, minced garlic, dried oregano, salt, and black pepper. Toss to coat the artichokes evenly.

4. Spoon the artichoke mixture over the chicken breasts, making sure to distribute the artichokes evenly.

5. Sprinkle the grated Parmesan cheese over the top of the chicken and artichokes.

6. Bake for 25•30 minutes, or until the chicken is cooked through and the internal temperature reaches 165°F (75°C).

7. Remove the baked chicken and artichokes from the oven and let it rest for 5 minutes before serving.

This baked chicken with artichokes dish is a great option for those with diabetes or high cholesterol. The chicken is a lean protein, and the artichokes provide fiber, vitamins, and minerals.

The Parmesan cheese adds flavor without too much saturated fat, and the lemon and garlic provide a bright, flavorful contrast to the chicken and artichokes.

Serve this dish with a side of roasted vegetables or a fresh salad for a complete, balanced meal. Enjoy this delicious and healthy baked chicken recipe!

30. Lentil and vegetable curry

Ingredient:

- 1 cup dry red lentils, rinsed
- 2 cups low•sodium vegetable broth
- 1 tbsp olive oil
- 1 onion, diced
- 3 garlic cloves, minced
- 1 tbsp grated fresh ginger
- 2 tsp curry powder
- 1 tsp ground cumin
- 1/2 tsp ground coriander
- 1/4 tsp cayenne pepper (optional)
- 1 (14 oz) can diced tomatoes, no salt added
- 2 cups chopped mixed vegetables (such as cauliflower, bell peppers, spinach)
- 1/4 tsp salt
- 1/4 tsp black pepper
- 2 tbsp chopped fresh cilantro (for garnish)

Instructions:

1. In a medium saucepan, combine the rinsed lentils and vegetable broth. Bring to a boil, then reduce heat and simmer for 15•20 minutes, until the lentils are tender.

2. In a large skillet or Dutch oven, heat the olive oil over medium heat. Add the diced onion and sauté for 3•4 minutes, until translucent.

3. Add the minced garlic and grated ginger to the skillet. Cook for 1 minute, until fragrant.

4. Stir in the curry powder, cumin, coriander, and cayenne (if using). Cook for 1 minute to toast the spices.

5. Add the diced tomatoes, chopped mixed vegetables, cooked lentils, salt, and black pepper. Stir to combine.

6. Reduce the heat to low and let the curry simmer for 10•15 minutes, until the vegetables are tender.

7. Remove the curry from heat and stir in the chopped fresh cilantro.

8. Serve the lentil and vegetable curry over steamed brown rice or quinoa.

This lentil and vegetable curry is a great option for those with diabetes or high cholesterol. It's high in fiber, protein, and nutrients, while being low in carbs and sodium. The variety of vegetables provides antioxidants and vitamins.

Adjust the amount of cayenne pepper to your desired level of spice. Enjoy this flavorful and healthy curry dish!

31. Turkey and avocado wrap

Ingredient:

- 4 whole wheat tortillas or wraps
- 8 oz sliced turkey breast
- 1 avocado, sliced
- 1 cup shredded romaine lettuce
- 2 tbsp plain Greek yogurt
- 1 tbsp Dijon mustard
- 1/4 tsp salt
- 1/4 tsp black pepper

Instructions:

1. In a small bowl, mix together the Greek yogurt, Dijon mustard, salt, and black pepper to make the dressing.

2. Lay the whole wheat tortillas or wraps on a flat surface. Spread the yogurt•mustard dressing evenly over each wrap.

3. Layer the sliced turkey breast, sliced avocado, and shredded romaine lettuce on the center of each wrap.

4. Fold the bottom of the wrap up over the filling, then fold in the sides and continue rolling up tightly to create a wrap.

5. Cut the wraps in half diagonally, if desired, and serve immediately.

This turkey and avocado wrap is a great option for those with diabetes or high cholesterol. It's high in protein from the turkey, healthy fats from the avocado, and fiber from the whole wheat wrap and lettuce.

The Greek yogurt•mustard dressing provides creaminess without the need for high•fat mayonnaise or cheese. You can adjust the amount of dressing to your preference.

This wrap makes a satisfying and nutritious lunch or light dinner. Pair it with a side salad or some fresh fruit for a complete, balanced meal.

32. Baked trout with almonds

Ingredient:

- 4 trout fillets (about 1 lb total)
- 2 tablespoons olive oil
- 1/2 cup sliced almonds
- 2 tablespoons unsalted butter, melted
- 2 tablespoons lemon juice
- 1 teaspoon lemon zest
- 1 teaspoon dried parsley
- Salt and black pepper to taste

Instructions:

1. Preheat your oven to 400°F. Line a baking sheet with parchment paper or foil.

2. Pat the trout fillets dry with paper towels and place them on the prepared baking sheet. Brush the fillets with the olive oil and season with salt and pepper.

3. In a small bowl, combine the sliced almonds, melted butter, lemon juice, lemon zest, and dried parsley. Stir to mix well.

4. Spoon the almond mixture evenly over the top of the trout fillets, pressing it down gently to help it adhere.

5. Bake the trout for 12•15 minutes, or until the fish flakes easily with a fork and the almonds are lightly golden.

6. Carefully transfer the baked trout fillets to a serving plate.

7. Serve the trout warm, garnished with any extra almond mixture from the baking sheet. Enjoy!

The combination of the tender, flaky trout with the crunchy, lemony almond topping makes this a delicious and easy baked fish dish. It's perfect for a quick weeknight meal or a special occasion.

33. Spinach and goat cheese stuffed chicken breast

Ingredient:

- 4 boneless, skinless chicken breasts
- 4 oz crumbled goat cheese
- 2 cups fresh spinach, chopped
- 2 cloves garlic, minced
- 1 tbsp olive oil
- 1/4 tsp salt
- 1/4 tsp black pepper

Instructions:

1. Preheat your oven to 400°F. Lightly grease a baking dish or line a baking sheet with parchment paper.

2. In a medium bowl, mix together the goat cheese, spinach, garlic, salt, and pepper until well combined.

3. Use a sharp knife to cut a pocket into the side of each chicken breast, being careful not to cut all the way through.

4. Stuff each chicken breast with about 2•3 tablespoons of the spinach and goat cheese mixture, pressing it into the pocket.

5. Place the stuffed chicken breasts in the prepared baking dish or on the baking sheet.

6. Drizzle the chicken with the olive oil, making sure to coat the tops and sides. Bake for 25•30 minutes, until the chicken is cooked through and the internal temperature reaches 165°F.

Tips for Diabetics and High Cholesterol:
• Chicken breast is a lean protein that is low in saturated fat.
• Goat cheese is lower in cholesterol and saturated fat compared to many other cheeses.
• Spinach is packed with vitamins, minerals, and fiber without adding a lot of carbs.
• Baking the chicken avoids the need for added oils or butter, keeping the dish low in unhealthy fats.

This stuffed chicken dish is a delicious and healthy option for those managing diabetes or high cholesterol. Serve it with a side of roasted vegetables for a complete and balanced meal. Enjoy!

34. Quinoa and black bean salad

Ingredient:

- 1 cup uncooked quinoa, rinsed
- 1 (15 oz) can black beans, drained and rinsed
- 1 cup diced cucumber
- 1 cup diced tomatoes
- 1/2 cup diced red onion
- 1/4 cup chopped fresh cilantro
- 2 tablespoons lime juice
- 1 tablespoon olive oil
- 1 teaspoon ground cumin
- 1/4 teaspoon salt
- 1/4 teaspoon black pepper

Instructions:

1. Cook the quinoa according to package instructions. Allow to cool completely.

2. In a large bowl, combine the cooked quinoa, black beans, cucumber, tomatoes, red onion, and cilantro.

3. In a small bowl, whisk together the lime juice, olive oil, cumin, salt, and pepper.

4. Pour the dressing over the quinoa and bean mixture and toss gently to coat everything evenly.

5. Refrigerate the salad for at least 30 minutes to allow the flavors to meld.

6. Serve chilled or at room temperature.

Tips:
- For extra protein, you can add grilled chicken or shrimp to this salad.
- Swap out the vegetables based on your preferences • bell peppers, corn, and avocado would also be great additions.
- This salad can be made ahead of time and keeps well in the refrigerator for 3•4 days.

This quinoa and black bean salad is packed with fiber, protein, and nutrients. It's a refreshing and healthy side dish or light main course. The combination of flavors and textures makes it a crowd•pleasing option. Enjoy!

35. Turkey and vegetable kebabs

Ingredient:

- 1 lb ground turkey
- 1 zucchini, cut into 1•inch pieces
- 1 red bell pepper, cut into 1•inch pieces
- 1 yellow onion, cut into 1•inch pieces
- 8 cherry tomatoes
- 2 tablespoons olive oil
- 1 teaspoon dried oregano
- 1/2 teaspoon garlic powder
- 1/4 teaspoon salt
- 1/4 teaspoon black pepper

Instructions:

1. Preheat your grill or grill pan to medium•high heat.

2. In a large bowl, combine the ground turkey, zucchini, bell pepper, onion, and cherry tomatoes. Drizzle with the olive oil and sprinkle with the oregano, garlic powder, salt, and pepper. Gently mix until everything is evenly coated.

3. Thread the turkey and vegetable pieces onto skewers, alternating the ingredients.

4. Grill the kebabs for 12•15 minutes, turning occasionally, until the turkey is cooked through and the vegetables are tender.

5. Serve the turkey and vegetable kebabs immediately, while hot.

Tips for Diabetics and High Cholesterol:
- Ground turkey is a lean protein that is lower in saturated fat compared to ground beef.
- The vegetables provide fiber, vitamins, and minerals without adding a lot of carbs or calories.
- Grilling the kebabs avoids the need for added oils or butter, keeping the dish low in unhealthy fats.
- You can adjust the seasoning to your taste preferences, avoiding high•sodium seasonings if needed.

This is a simple, healthy, and delicious meal that is perfect for those watching their blood sugar or cholesterol levels. Enjoy!

36. Baked sweet potato fries

Ingredient:

- 2 lbs sweet potatoes, peeled and cut into 1/2•inch thick fry shapes
- 2 tablespoons olive oil
- 1 teaspoon paprika
- 1 teaspoon garlic powder
- 1/2 teaspoon salt
- 1/4 teaspoon black pepper

Instructions:

1. Preheat your oven to 400°F. Line a large baking sheet with parchment paper.

2. In a large bowl, toss the sweet potato fry shapes with the olive oil, paprika, garlic powder, salt, and pepper until evenly coated.

3. Spread the seasoned sweet potato fries in a single layer on the prepared baking sheet, making sure they are not touching each other.

4. Bake for 20 minutes, then flip the fries and bake for an additional 15•20 minutes, until they are crispy and lightly browned.

5. Remove the baked sweet potato fries from the oven and let them cool for 5 minutes before serving.

Tips:
- Cut the sweet potatoes into even thickness so they cook evenly.

- Soak the cut fries in cold water for 30 minutes before baking to remove excess starch, then pat them very dry before tossing with oil and seasonings.

- For extra crispiness, bake the fries on the top oven rack.

Serve the baked sweet potato fries warm, seasoned with additional salt if desired. They make a delicious, healthier alternative to regular french fries. Enjoy!

37. Grilled chicken and vegetable skewers

Ingredient:

- 2 tablespoons olive oil
- 2 tablespoons lemon juice
- 1 teaspoon dried oregano
- 1/2 teaspoon garlic powder
- 1/4 teaspoon salt
- 1/4 teaspoon black pepper

- 1 lb boneless, skinless chicken breasts, cut into 1•inch cubes
- 1 red bell pepper, cut into 1•inch pieces
- 1 zucchini, cut into 1•inch pieces
- 1 red onion, cut into 1•inch pieces
- 8 oz mushrooms, halved

Instructions:

1. Preheat your grill or grill pan to medium•high heat.

2. In a large bowl, combine the cubed chicken, bell pepper, zucchini, onion, and mushrooms.

3. In a small bowl, whisk together the olive oil, lemon juice, oregano, garlic powder, salt, and pepper.

4. Pour the marinade over the chicken and vegetables and toss to coat everything evenly.

5. Thread the marinated chicken and vegetables onto skewers, alternating the ingredients.

6. Grill the skewers for 12•15 minutes, turning occasionally, until the chicken is cooked through and the vegetables are tender. Serve the grilled chicken and vegetable skewers immediately, while hot.

Tips:
- Soak wooden skewers in water for 30 minutes before using to prevent them from burning.
- You can use any combination of your favorite vegetables, such as cherry tomatoes, eggplant, or asparagus.
- For extra flavor, you can baste the skewers with any leftover marinade during the last few minutes of grilling.

This grilled chicken and vegetable skewer recipe is a healthy, easy•to•make meal that's perfect for summer. The combination of lean protein and fresh produce makes it a great option for a balanced and delicious dinner. Enjoy!

38. Tofu stir•fry with broccoli and bell peppers

Ingredient:

- 1 block (14 oz) extra•firm tofu, pressed and cubed
- 2 tablespoons sesame oil
- 2 cloves garlic, minced
- 1 tablespoon grated fresh ginger
- 1 head broccoli, cut into florets
- 1 red bell pepper, sliced
- 1 yellow bell pepper, sliced
- 3 tablespoons low•sodium soy sauce
- 2 tablespoons rice vinegar
- 1 tablespoon honey
- 1 teaspoon cornstarch
- Salt and pepper to taste
- Chopped green onions and sesame seeds for garnish (optional)

Instructions:

1. In a large skillet or wok, heat the sesame oil over medium•high heat. Add the cubed tofu and cook for 5•7 minutes, turning occasionally, until lightly browned on all sides. Transfer the tofu to a plate.

2. In the same skillet, add the garlic and ginger. Cook for 1 minute until fragrant.

3. Add the broccoli florets and bell pepper slices. Stir•fry for 5•7 minutes, until the vegetables are crisp•tender.

4. In a small bowl, whisk together the soy sauce, rice vinegar, honey, and cornstarch.

5. Add the cooked tofu back to the skillet with the vegetables. Pour in the soy sauce mixture and toss everything together. Cook for 2•3 minutes, until the sauce has thickened.

6. Season with salt and pepper to taste.

7. Serve the tofu stir•fry hot, garnished with chopped green onions and sesame seeds if desired. Enjoy!

This tofu stir•fry is a delicious and nutritious vegetarian meal. The combination of crisp•tender vegetables and flavorful tofu makes it a satisfying and balanced dish. Adjust the spices and seasonings to your taste preferences.

39. Zucchini noodles with pesto

Ingredient:

- 3•4 medium zucchinis, spiralized or julienned into noodles
- 1/2 cup basil pesto (store•bought or homemade)
- 1/4 cup grated Parmesan cheese
- 2 tablespoons toasted pine nuts
- Salt and pepper to taste

For the Basil Pesto:
- 2 cups fresh basil leaves
- 1/4 cup pine nuts
- 2 cloves garlic
- 1/4 cup olive oil
- 1/4 cup grated Parmesan cheese
- Salt and pepper to taste

Instructions:
For the Pesto:
1. In a food processor, combine the basil, pine nuts, and garlic. Pulse until finely chopped.

2. With the processor running, slowly drizzle in the olive oil until a smooth pesto forms.

3. Stir in the Parmesan cheese and season with salt and pepper to taste.

For the Zucchini Noodles:
1. Use a spiralizer, julienne peeler, or mandoline to cut the zucchinis into long, thin noodles.

2. In a large bowl, toss the zucchini noodles with the basil pesto until evenly coated.

3. Top with the grated Parmesan cheese and toasted pine nuts.

4. Season with salt and pepper to taste.

To Serve:
Serve the zucchini noodles with pesto immediately, while the noodles are still crisp. You can also let the noodles sit for 5•10 minutes to allow the flavors to meld.

This dish is a delicious, low•carb alternative to traditional pasta. The fresh basil pesto complements the zucchini noodles perfectly. Enjoy!

40. Cauliflower rice with mixed vegetables

Ingredient:

- 1 head of cauliflower, cut into florets
- 1 tablespoon olive oil
- 1 onion, diced
- 2 cloves garlic, minced
- 1 cup diced carrots
- 1 cup diced zucchini
- 1 cup frozen peas
- 2 tablespoons low•sodium soy sauce or tamari
- 1 teaspoon ground ginger
- 1/4 teaspoon red pepper flakes (optional)
- Salt and pepper to taste
- Chopped fresh parsley for garnish (optional)

Instructions:

1. In a food processor, pulse the cauliflower florets until they resemble the size and texture of rice. Set aside.

2. In a large skillet or wok, heat the olive oil over medium•high heat. Add the diced onion and sauté for 3•4 minutes until translucent.

3. Add the minced garlic and sauté for 1 minute until fragrant.

4. Stir in the diced carrots, zucchini, and frozen peas. Cook for 5•7 minutes, until the vegetables are tender•crisp.

5. Add the cauliflower rice to the skillet and stir to combine. Cook for 3•5 minutes, until the cauliflower rice is heated through.

6. Drizzle the soy sauce or tamari over the cauliflower rice and vegetables. Sprinkle in the ground ginger and red pepper flakes (if using). Toss everything together until well mixed.

7. Season with salt and pepper to taste. Serve the cauliflower rice and vegetable mixture warm, garnished with chopped fresh parsley if desired.

This cauliflower rice dish is a delicious, low•carb alternative to traditional rice. The mix of fresh vegetables adds color, texture, and plenty of nutrients. It's a versatile and healthy side dish or meatless main course. Enjoy!

41. Greek salad with grilled chicken

Ingredient:

For the Salad:
- 1 head romaine lettuce, chopped
- 1 cucumber, diced
- 1 pint cherry tomatoes, halved
- 1 red onion, thinly sliced
- 1 cup crumbled feta cheese
- 1/2 cup Kalamata olives, pitted and halved

For the Grilled Chicken:
- 4 boneless, skinless chicken breasts
- 2 tablespoons olive oil
- 1 teaspoon dried oregano
- 1/2 teaspoon garlic powder
- Salt and pepper to taste

For the Dressing:
- 1/4 cup olive oil
- 2 tablespoons red wine vinegar
- 1 tablespoon lemon juice
- 1 teaspoon Dijon mustard
- 1 clove garlic, minced
- 1/2 teaspoon dried oregano
- 1/4 teaspoon salt
- 1/4 teaspoon black pepper

Instructions:

1. Preheat your grill or grill pan to medium•high heat.

2. In a small bowl, combine the olive oil, oregano, garlic powder, salt, and pepper. Rub the mixture all over the chicken breasts.

3. Grill the chicken for 5•7 minutes per side, or until cooked through. Let rest for 5 minutes, then slice or chop the chicken.

4. In a large salad bowl, combine the chopped romaine, cucumber, cherry tomatoes, red onion, feta cheese, and Kalamata olives.

5. In a small bowl, whisk together the dressing ingredients: olive oil, red wine vinegar, lemon juice, Dijon mustard, garlic, oregano, salt, and pepper.

6. Add the grilled chicken to the salad and drizzle the dressing over the top. Toss gently to coat. Serve the Greek salad with grilled chicken immediately.

This Greek salad with grilled chicken is a healthy, flavorful, and satisfying meal. The combination of fresh vegetables, tangy feta, and juicy chicken makes it a delicious and nutritious option. Enjoy!

42. Tuna and white bean salad

Ingredient:

- 2 (5 oz) cans tuna, drained and flaked
- 1 (15 oz) can white beans, drained and rinsed
- 1/2 cup diced celery
- 1/4 cup diced red onion
- 2 tablespoons chopped fresh parsley
- 2 tablespoons lemon juice
- 1 tablespoon olive oil
- 1 teaspoon Dijon mustard
- 1/4 teaspoon salt
- 1/4 teaspoon black pepper

Instructions:

1. In a medium bowl, combine the flaked tuna, white beans, celery, red onion, and parsley.

2. In a small bowl, whisk together the lemon juice, olive oil, Dijon mustard, salt, and pepper.

3. Pour the dressing over the tuna and bean mixture and stir gently to coat everything evenly.

4. Refrigerate the salad for at least 30 minutes to allow the flavors to meld.

5. Serve chilled or at room temperature.

Tips:
- You can use any type of canned white beans, such as cannellini or navy beans.

- For extra crunch, add some diced cucumber or bell pepper.

- Swap the parsley for other fresh herbs like dill or basil.

- This salad can be made ahead of time and keeps well in the refrigerator for 3•4 days.

This tuna and white bean salad is a simple, healthy, and delicious option for a light lunch or side dish. The combination of protein•rich tuna, fiber•filled beans, and fresh vegetables makes it a nutritious and satisfying meal. Enjoy!

43. Roasted Brussels sprouts with walnuts

Ingredient:

- 1 lb Brussels sprouts, trimmed and halved
- 2 tablespoons olive oil
- 1/2 teaspoon salt
- 1/4 teaspoon black pepper
- 1/2 cup chopped walnuts
- 2 tablespoons balsamic glaze (or balsamic vinegar)
- 2 tablespoons grated Parmesan cheese (optional)

Instructions:

1. Preheat your oven to 400°F. Line a baking sheet with parchment paper.

2. In a large bowl, toss the Brussels sprout halves with the olive oil, salt, and pepper until evenly coated.

3. Spread the Brussels sprouts in a single layer on the prepared baking sheet.

4. Roast the Brussels sprouts for 18•22 minutes, tossing halfway, until they are tender and lightly browned.

5. Remove the roasted Brussels sprouts from the oven and transfer them to a serving bowl.

6. Add the chopped walnuts and drizzle the balsamic glaze over the top. Toss gently to combine.

7. If desired, sprinkle the roasted Brussels sprouts with the grated Parmesan cheese.

8. Serve the roasted Brussels sprouts with walnuts warm.

Tips:
- For extra flavor, you can roast the walnuts along with the Brussels sprouts for 5•7 minutes.
- Swap the balsamic glaze for balsamic vinegar if you prefer a tangier flavor.
- This dish can be served as a side or as a main course with a protein like grilled chicken or salmon.

The combination of tender, caramelized Brussels sprouts, crunchy walnuts, and tangy balsamic glaze makes this a delicious and nutritious side dish. Enjoy!

44. Baked salmon with dill sauce

Ingredient:

For the Dill Sauce:
- 1/2 cup plain Greek yogurt
- 2 tablespoons chopped fresh dill
- 1 tablespoon lemon juice
- 1 teaspoon Dijon mustard
- 1 clove garlic, minced
- 1/4 teaspoon salt
- 1/4 teaspoon black pepper

For the Salmon:
- 4 (6 oz) salmon fillets
- 1 tablespoon olive oil
- 1 teaspoon lemon zest
- Salt and pepper to taste

Instructions:

1. Preheat your oven to 400°F. Line a baking sheet with parchment paper or foil.

2. Place the salmon fillets on the prepared baking sheet. Drizzle with the olive oil and sprinkle with the lemon zest, salt, and pepper.

3. Bake the salmon for 12•15 minutes, or until it flakes easily with a fork and reaches an internal temperature of 145°F.

For the Dill Sauce:
1. In a small bowl, whisk together the Greek yogurt, chopped dill, lemon juice, Dijon mustard, garlic, salt, and pepper.

2. Serve the baked salmon warm, with the dill sauce spooned over the top or on the side for dipping.

Tips:
- You can use fresh or dried dill in the sauce. Adjust the amount to your taste preference.
- For extra flavor, you can also add a squeeze of lemon juice over the salmon before baking.
- Serve the salmon and dill sauce with roasted vegetables or a fresh salad for a complete, healthy meal.

This baked salmon with dill sauce is a simple yet elegant dish that's perfect for a weeknight dinner or special occasion. The cool, creamy dill sauce complements the rich, flaky salmon beautifully. Enjoy!

45. Shrimp and avocado salad

Ingredient:

- 1 lb cooked shrimp, peeled and deveined
- 2 avocados, diced
- 1 cup cherry tomatoes, halved
- 1/2 red onion, thinly sliced
- 1/4 cup chopped fresh cilantro
- 2 tablespoons lime juice
- 1 tablespoon olive oil
- 1/2 teaspoon salt
- 1/4 teaspoon black pepper

Instructions:

1. In a large bowl, gently combine the cooked shrimp, diced avocado, cherry tomatoes, red onion, and chopped cilantro.

2. In a small bowl, whisk together the lime juice, olive oil, salt, and black pepper to make the dressing.

3. Pour the dressing over the shrimp and avocado salad and toss gently to coat everything evenly.

4. Refrigerate the salad for at least 30 minutes to allow the flavors to meld.

5. Serve the shrimp and avocado salad chilled or at room temperature.

Tips:
- You can use cooked and peeled shrimp or grilled shrimp for this recipe.
- For extra crunch, add some chopped romaine lettuce or baby spinach.
- Swap the cilantro for fresh parsley or basil if desired.
- This salad can be made ahead of time and keeps well in the refrigerator for 2•3 days.

This shrimp and avocado salad is a refreshing and nutritious dish. The combination of tender shrimp, creamy avocado, juicy tomatoes, and tangy lime dressing makes it a delicious and satisfying meal or side. Enjoy!

46. Eggplant rollatini

Ingredient:

- 1 large eggplant, sliced lengthwise into 1/4•inch thick slices
- 2 tablespoons olive oil
- 1 cup part•skim ricotta cheese
- 1/2 cup grated mozzarella cheese
- 1/4 cup grated Parmesan cheese
- 1 egg, lightly beaten
- 2 cloves garlic, minced
- 1/4 cup chopped fresh basil
- 1/4 teaspoon salt
- 1/4 teaspoon black pepper
- 1 cup marinara sauce
- 2 tablespoons grated Parmesan cheese for topping

Instructions:

1. Preheat your oven to 375°F. Lightly grease a 9x13 inch baking dish.

2. Brush the eggplant slices on both sides with the olive oil. Place them in a single layer on a baking sheet.

3. Bake the eggplant slices for 10•12 minutes, flipping halfway, until they are tender and pliable.

4. In a medium bowl, mix together the ricotta, mozzarella, 1/4 cup Parmesan, egg, garlic, basil, salt, and pepper until well combined.

5. Spread about 2•3 tablespoons of the ricotta mixture onto the end of each eggplant slice. Carefully roll up the eggplant and place seam•side down in the prepared baking dish.

6. Pour the marinara sauce evenly over the eggplant rollatini. Sprinkle the remaining 2 tablespoons of Parmesan cheese on top.

7. Bake for 20•25 minutes, until the cheese is melted and bubbly.

8. Let the eggplant rollatini cool for 5 minutes before serving.

Serve the eggplant rollatini warm, garnished with additional fresh basil if desired. This dish makes a delicious vegetarian main course or side dish. Enjoy!

47. Spinach and mushroom stuffed chicken breast

Ingredient:

- 4 boneless, skinless chicken breasts
- 8 oz cremini or button mushrooms, finely chopped
- 2 cups fresh spinach, chopped
- 2 cloves garlic, minced
- 1/4 cup grated Parmesan cheese
- 2 tablespoons cream cheese, softened
- 1/4 teaspoon salt
- 1/4 teaspoon black pepper
- 1 tablespoon olive oil

Instructions:

1. Preheat your oven to 400°F. Lightly grease a baking dish or line a baking sheet with parchment paper.

2. In a skillet over medium heat, sauté the chopped mushrooms until they release their moisture and start to brown, about 5•7 minutes. Add the spinach and garlic and cook for 2•3 minutes more, until the spinach is wilted. Remove from heat and let cool slightly.

3. In a medium bowl, mix together the sautéed mushroom•spinach mixture, Parmesan cheese, cream cheese, salt, and pepper until well combined.

4. Use a sharp knife to cut a pocket into the side of each chicken breast, being careful not to cut all the way through.

5. Stuff each chicken breast with about 1/4 of the spinach and mushroom filling, pressing it into the pocket.

6. Place the stuffed chicken breasts in the prepared baking dish or on the baking sheet. Drizzle the tops with the olive oil.

7. Bake for 25•30 minutes, until the chicken is cooked through and the internal temperature reaches 165°F.

8. Let the stuffed chicken breasts rest for 5 minutes before serving.

This spinach and mushroom stuffed chicken breast is a delicious and healthy main dish. The savory filling complements the juicy chicken perfectly. Serve it with a side of roasted vegetables or a fresh salad for a complete meal. Enjoy!

48. Chickpea and vegetable curry

Ingredient:

- 2 tablespoons olive oil
- 1 onion, diced
- 3 cloves garlic, minced
- 1 tablespoon grated fresh ginger
- 2 teaspoons garam masala
- 1 teaspoon ground cumin
- 1 teaspoon ground coriander
- 1/2 teaspoon turmeric
- 1/4 teaspoon cayenne pepper (or to taste)
- 1 (15 oz) can chickpeas, drained and rinsed
- 1 (14 oz) can diced tomatoes
- 1 cup vegetable broth
- 1 medium potato, peeled and diced
- 1 cup cauliflower florets
- 1 cup frozen peas
- 1 cup spinach leaves
- Salt and pepper to taste
- Chopped cilantro for garnish

Instructions:

1. In a large skillet or pot, heat the olive oil over medium heat. Add the onion and sauté for 5 minutes until translucent.

2. Add the garlic and ginger and sauté for 1 minute until fragrant.

3. Stir in the garam masala, cumin, coriander, turmeric, and cayenne. Cook for 1 minute to toast the spices.

4. Add the chickpeas, diced tomatoes, vegetable broth, potato, cauliflower, and peas. Bring to a simmer.

5. Reduce heat to medium•low and let the curry simmer for 15•20 minutes, until the vegetables are tender.

6. Stir in the spinach leaves and cook for 2•3 minutes until wilted.

7. Season with salt and pepper to taste.

8. Serve the chickpea and vegetable curry warm, garnished with chopped cilantro. Enjoy!

This curry is packed with protein from the chickpeas and plenty of veggies. It's a hearty, flavorful meatless meal. Serve it over basmati rice or with naan bread.

49. Turkey and quinoa stuffed bell peppers

Ingredient:

- 4 bell peppers, halved lengthwise and seeds removed
- 1 lb ground turkey
- 1 cup cooked quinoa
- 1 small onion, diced
- 2 cloves garlic, minced
- 1 (14.5 oz) can diced tomatoes
- 1 teaspoon dried oregano
- 1/2 teaspoon ground cumin
- 1/4 teaspoon red pepper flakes (optional)
- 1/2 cup shredded part•skim mozzarella cheese
- Salt and black pepper to taste

Instructions:

1. Preheat your oven to 375°F. Lightly grease a baking dish or line it with parchment paper.

2. Arrange the bell pepper halves in the prepared baking dish.

3. In a large skillet over medium heat, cook the ground turkey, breaking it up with a wooden spoon, until no longer pink, about 5•7 minutes.

4. Add the diced onion and garlic to the skillet and cook for 2•3 minutes until fragrant.

5. Stir in the cooked quinoa, diced tomatoes, oregano, cumin, and red pepper flakes (if using). Season with salt and black pepper to taste.

6. Spoon the turkey and quinoa mixture evenly into the bell pepper halves. Top each stuffed pepper with a sprinkle of the shredded mozzarella cheese.

7. Bake the stuffed peppers for 25•30 minutes, until the peppers are tender and the cheese is melted and bubbly. Serve the turkey and quinoa stuffed bell peppers warm.

Tips for Diabetics and High Cholesterol:
- Ground turkey is a lean protein that is lower in saturated fat compared to ground beef.
- Quinoa is a high•fiber, gluten•free grain that provides complex carbs and protein.
- The bell peppers and tomatoes add fiber, vitamins, and minerals without a lot of carbs or calories.
- The small amount of mozzarella cheese keeps the dish low in saturated fat and cholesterol

50. Baked eggplant Parmesan

Ingredient:

- 2 medium eggplants, sliced into 1/2•inch thick rounds
- 2 cups marinara sauce
- 1 cup shredded mozzarella cheese
- 1/2 cup grated Parmesan cheese
- 1/4 cup all•purpose flour
- 2 eggs, beaten
- 1 cup breadcrumbs
- 2 tablespoons olive oil
- 1 teaspoon dried oregano
- 1/2 teaspoon garlic powder
- Salt and pepper to taste

Instructions:

1. Preheat your oven to 375°F. Lightly grease a 9x13 inch baking dish.

2. Set up a breading station with three shallow dishes: one with the flour, one with the beaten eggs, and one with the breadcrumbs mixed with the oregano, garlic powder, salt, and pepper.

3. Dip the eggplant slices first in the flour, then the egg, and finally the breadcrumb mixture, coating both sides.

4. Arrange the breaded eggplant slices in a single layer on the prepared baking dish. Drizzle the tops with the olive oil.

5. Bake the eggplant for 20•25 minutes, flipping halfway, until golden brown and crispy.

6. Remove the baked eggplant from the oven and top each slice with a spoonful of marinara sauce, followed by the mozzarella and Parmesan cheeses.

7. Return the dish to the oven and bake for an additional 10•15 minutes, until the cheese is melted and bubbly.

8. Let the baked eggplant Parmesan cool for 5 minutes before serving.

Serve the eggplant Parmesan warm, garnished with fresh basil or parsley if desired. This dish makes a delicious vegetarian main course or side. Enjoy!

51. Grilled shrimp with avocado salsa

Ingredient:

For the Shrimp:
- 1 lb large shrimp, peeled and deveined
- 1 tablespoon olive oil
- 1 teaspoon chili powder
- 1/2 teaspoon garlic powder
- 1/4 teaspoon salt
- 1/4 teaspoon black pepper

For the Avocado Salsa:
- 1 ripe avocado, diced
- 1/2 cup diced tomatoes
- 1/4 cup diced red onion
- 2 tablespoons chopped fresh cilantro
- 1 tablespoon lime juice
- 1/4 teaspoon salt

Instructions:

1. Preheat your grill or grill pan to medium•high heat.

2. In a medium bowl, toss the shrimp with the olive oil, chili powder, garlic powder, salt, and pepper until evenly coated.

3. Thread the seasoned shrimp onto skewers, if desired.

4. Grill the shrimp for 2•3 minutes per side, until they are opaque and cooked through.

5. While the shrimp are grilling, prepare the avocado salsa. In a small bowl, gently mix together the diced avocado, tomatoes, red onion, cilantro, lime juice, and salt.

6. Serve the grilled shrimp warm, topped with the avocado salsa.

Tips for Diabetics and High Cholesterol:
- Shrimp is a lean protein that is low in saturated fat and high in beneficial omega•3 fatty acids.

- Avocado provides healthy monounsaturated fats, fiber, and antioxidants without adding a lot of carbs or cholesterol.

- The fresh salsa adds flavor without the need for high•sodium sauces or dressings.

- Grilling the shrimp avoids the need for added oils or butter, keeping the dish low in unhealthy fats.

This grilled shrimp with avocado salsa is a delicious and nutritious option for those managing diabetes or high cholesterol. Enjoy!

52. Cauliflower crust pizza with spinach and feta

Ingredient:

For the Toppings:
- 1 cup fresh spinach, chopped
- 1/2 cup crumbled feta cheese
- 1/4 cup shredded part•skim mozzarella cheese
- 1/4 cup diced tomatoes
- 1 tablespoon olive oil

For the Cauliflower Crust:
- 1 head of cauliflower, riced (about 3 cups riced cauliflower)
- 1 egg, beaten
- 1/4 cup grated Parmesan cheese
- 1/4 teaspoon garlic powder
- 1/4 teaspoon dried oregano
- 1/4 teaspoon salt

Instructions:

1. Preheat your oven to 400°F. Line a baking sheet with parchment paper.

2. To make the cauliflower crust, place the riced cauliflower in a microwave•safe bowl and microwave for 5•7 minutes, until tender. Allow to cool slightly.

3. Transfer the cooked cauliflower to a clean kitchen towel and squeeze out as much moisture as possible.

4. In a bowl, mix the squeezed cauliflower, beaten egg, Parmesan, garlic powder, oregano, and salt until well combined.

5. Press the cauliflower mixture onto the prepared baking sheet, forming a thin, even crust.

6. Bake the cauliflower crust for 20•25 minutes, until golden brown.

7. Remove the crust from the oven and top with the chopped spinach, crumbled feta, shredded mozzarella, and diced tomatoes.

8. Drizzle the pizza with the olive oil. Bake the pizza for an additional 10•15 minutes, until the cheese is melted and bubbly. Let the pizza cool for 5 minutes before slicing and serving.

Tips for Diabetics and High Cholesterol:
- Cauliflower is a low•carb, high•fiber vegetable that makes a great pizza crust alternative.
- Spinach and feta provide nutrients and flavor without adding a lot of saturated fat or cholesterol.
- The small amount of mozzarella cheese and olive oil keeps the dish low in unhealthy fats.

53. Greek yogurt with nuts and seeds

Ingredient:

- 1 cup plain Greek yogurt
- 2 tablespoons chopped walnuts
- 2 tablespoons chopped almonds
- 1 tablespoon chia seeds
- 1 tablespoon ground flaxseeds
- 1 tablespoon unsweetened shredded coconut
- 1 teaspoon honey (optional)
- 1/4 teaspoon ground cinnamon

Instructions:

1. In a medium bowl, combine the plain Greek yogurt, chopped walnuts, chopped almonds, chia seeds, ground flaxseeds, and unsweetened shredded coconut.

2. If desired, drizzle the yogurt mixture with 1 teaspoon of honey and sprinkle with the ground cinnamon.

3. Stir everything together until well combined.

4. Serve the Greek yogurt with nuts and seeds immediately, or cover and refrigerate until ready to enjoy.

Tips:
- Use plain, unsweetened Greek yogurt to keep the sugar content low.
- Feel free to adjust the amounts of nuts and seeds based on your preferences.
- Other great additions could include fresh berries, sliced bananas, or a sprinkle of granola.
- This makes a satisfying and nutritious breakfast, snack, or dessert.

This Greek yogurt with nuts and seeds is a delicious and healthy option that's packed with protein, healthy fats, fiber, and essential vitamins and minerals. It's a great choice for those with diabetes or high cholesterol, as the combination of nutrient•dense ingredients can help support overall health. Enjoy!

54. Baked chicken with lemon and capers

Ingredient:

- 4 boneless, skinless chicken breasts
- 2 tablespoons olive oil
- 2 tablespoons lemon juice
- 2 tablespoons capers, drained
- 1 teaspoon lemon zest
- 1 teaspoon dried oregano
- 1/4 teaspoon salt
- 1/4 teaspoon black pepper

Instructions:

1. Preheat your oven to 400°F. Lightly grease a baking dish or line a baking sheet with parchment paper.

2. Place the chicken breasts in the prepared baking dish or on the baking sheet.

3. In a small bowl, whisk together the olive oil, lemon juice, capers, lemon zest, oregano, salt, and pepper.

4. Pour the lemon•caper mixture over the chicken, making sure to coat the breasts evenly.

5. Bake the chicken for 25•30 minutes, or until it reaches an internal temperature of 165°F and the juices run clear.

6. Serve the baked chicken with lemon and capers warm.

Tips for Diabetics and High Cholesterol:
- Chicken breast is a lean protein that is low in saturated fat.
- Lemon and capers add flavor without the need for high•sodium seasonings or sauces.
- Baking the chicken avoids the need for added oils or butter, keeping the dish low in unhealthy fats.
- Serve the chicken with roasted vegetables or a fresh salad for a complete, balanced meal.

This baked chicken with lemon and capers is a delicious and healthy option for those managing diabetes or high cholesterol. The bright, tangy flavors complement the juicy chicken perfectly. Enjoy!

55. Lentil and spinach soup

Ingredient:

- 1 tablespoon olive oil
- 1 onion, diced
- 3 cloves garlic, minced
- 1 cup dried brown or green lentils, rinsed
- 4 cups low•sodium vegetable or chicken broth
- 1 (14.5 oz) can diced tomatoes
- 1 teaspoon dried thyme
- 1/2 teaspoon ground cumin
- 1/4 teaspoon red pepper flakes (optional)
- 4 cups fresh spinach, chopped
- Salt and black pepper to taste

Instructions:

1. In a large pot or Dutch oven, heat the olive oil over medium heat. Add the diced onion and sauté for 5 minutes until translucent.

2. Add the minced garlic and sauté for 1 minute until fragrant.

3. Stir in the rinsed lentils, vegetable or chicken broth, diced tomatoes, thyme, cumin, and red pepper flakes (if using). Bring the soup to a boil.

4. Reduce the heat to medium•low and let the soup simmer for 20•25 minutes, until the lentils are tender.

5. Stir in the chopped fresh spinach and cook for 2•3 minutes more, until the spinach is wilted. Season the soup with salt and black pepper to taste.

Tips for Diabetics and High Cholesterol:
- Lentils are a great source of plant•based protein, fiber, and complex carbs, making them a diabetes•friendly ingredient.
- Spinach is packed with vitamins, minerals, and antioxidants without adding a lot of carbs or calories.
- Using low•sodium broth and avoiding high•sodium seasonings helps keep the dish heart•healthy.
- This soup is naturally low in saturated fat and cholesterol, making it a great option for those with high cholesterol.

Serve this nourishing Lentil and Spinach Soup warm, with a sprinkle of grated Parmesan cheese or a slice of whole•grain bread on the side. Enjoy!

56. Turkey and vegetable stir•fry with brown rice

Ingredient:

- 1 lb ground turkey
- 2 tablespoons low•sodium soy sauce
- 1 tablespoon rice vinegar
- 1 teaspoon sesame oil
- 1 teaspoon grated fresh ginger
- 1 clove garlic, minced
- 2 cups mixed vegetables (such as broccoli, bell peppers, snow peas, carrots)
- 2 cups cooked brown rice
- 2 tablespoons chopped green onions (optional)
- Salt and pepper to taste

Instructions:

1. In a large skillet or wok, cook the ground turkey over medium•high heat, breaking it up with a wooden spoon, until no longer pink, about 5•7 minutes.

2. In a small bowl, whisk together the soy sauce, rice vinegar, sesame oil, ginger, and garlic.

3. Add the mixed vegetables to the skillet with the cooked turkey. Pour the soy sauce mixture over the top and stir to coat everything evenly.

4. Cook the stir•fry for 5•7 minutes, stirring frequently, until the vegetables are tender•crisp.

5. Serve the turkey and vegetable stir•fry over the cooked brown rice. Garnish with chopped green onions, if desired. Season with salt and pepper to taste.

Tips for Diabetics and High Cholesterol:

- Ground turkey is a lean protein that is lower in saturated fat compared to ground beef.

- Brown rice is a whole grain that provides complex carbs, fiber, and nutrients.

- The vegetables add fiber, vitamins, and minerals without a lot of carbs or calories.

- The low•sodium soy sauce and minimal oil keep the dish heart•healthy.

This turkey and vegetable stir•fry with brown rice is a delicious and nutritious meal that's perfect for those managing diabetes or high cholesterol. Enjoy!

57. Baked trout with lemon and herbs

Ingredient:

- 4 trout fillets (about 1 lb total)
- 2 tablespoons olive oil
- 2 tablespoons lemon juice
- 1 tablespoon chopped fresh parsley
- 1 tablespoon chopped fresh dill
- 2 cloves garlic, minced
- 1/4 teaspoon salt
- 1/4 teaspoon black pepper

Instructions:

1. Preheat your oven to 400°F. Lightly grease a baking dish or line a baking sheet with parchment paper.

2. In a small bowl, whisk together the olive oil, lemon juice, parsley, dill, garlic, salt, and pepper.

3. Place the trout fillets in the prepared baking dish or on the baking sheet. Spoon the lemon•herb mixture evenly over the top of the fish, making sure to coat all the fillets.

4. Bake the trout for 15•18 minutes, or until it flakes easily with a fork and reaches an internal temperature of 145°F.

Tips for Diabetics and High Cholesterol:

• Trout is a lean, heart•healthy fish that is low in saturated fat and high in omega•3 fatty acids.

• The lemon, herbs, and garlic add flavor without the need for high•sodium seasonings or sauces.

• Baking the trout avoids the need for added oils or butter, keeping the dish low in unhealthy fats.

• Serve the baked trout with roasted vegetables or a fresh salad for a complete, balanced meal.

This baked trout with lemon and herbs is a delicious and nutritious option for those managing diabetes or high cholesterol. The bright, flavorful topping complements the mild, flaky fish perfectly. Enjoy!

58. Spinach and feta stuffed turkey meatballs

Ingredient:

- 1 lb ground turkey
- 1 cup fresh spinach, chopped
- 1/2 cup crumbled feta cheese
- 1/4 cup whole wheat breadcrumbs
- 1 egg, lightly beaten
- 2 cloves garlic, minced
- 1 tsp dried oregano
- 1/4 tsp salt
- 1/4 tsp black pepper

Instructions:

1. Preheat oven to 400°F. Line a baking sheet with parchment paper.

2. In a large bowl, combine the ground turkey, spinach, feta, breadcrumbs, egg, garlic, oregano, salt, and pepper. Mix well until all ingredients are evenly distributed.

3. Scoop out about 2 tablespoons of the mixture and roll it into a ball. Place the meatball on the prepared baking sheet. Repeat with the remaining mixture.

4. Bake for 20•25 minutes, or until the meatballs are cooked through and no longer pink in the center.

5. Serve warm, either on their own or with a side of roasted vegetables or a salad.

These meatballs are a great source of protein from the turkey, and the spinach and feta provide important nutrients while keeping the cholesterol and carbohydrates low. The whole wheat breadcrumbs also add some fiber. Enjoy!

59. Quinoa and black bean stuffed bell peppers

Ingredient:

- 4 bell peppers (any color)
- 1 cup cooked quinoa
- 1 (15 oz) can black beans, rinsed and drained
- 1/2 cup diced onion
- 2 cloves garlic, minced
- 1 tsp ground cumin
- 1 tsp chili powder
- 1/4 tsp salt
- 1/4 tsp black pepper
- 1/2 cup shredded low•fat cheddar cheese (optional)

Instructions:

1. Preheat oven to 375°F. Cut the tops off the bell peppers and remove the seeds and membranes. Place the peppers in a baking dish.

2. In a medium bowl, combine the cooked quinoa, black beans, onion, garlic, cumin, chili powder, salt, and pepper. Mix well.

3. Stuff the quinoa and black bean mixture into the hollowed•out bell peppers, packing it in tightly.

4. If using the cheese, sprinkle it evenly over the tops of the stuffed peppers.

5. Bake for 25•30 minutes, until the peppers are tender and the filling is hot.

6. Serve the stuffed peppers warm.

These stuffed peppers are a great source of fiber, protein, and complex carbohydrates from the quinoa and black beans. The bell peppers provide vitamins A and C. This dish is a healthy and satisfying meal for those with diabetes or high cholesterol.

60. Turkey and avocado salad

Ingredient:

- 2 cups cooked turkey breast, diced
- 1 avocado, diced
- 1/2 cup diced celery
- 1/4 cup diced red onion
- 2 tbsp chopped fresh parsley
- 2 tbsp olive oil
- 1 tbsp lemon juice
- 1/4 tsp salt
- 1/4 tsp black pepper

Instructions:

1. In a large bowl, combine the diced turkey, avocado, celery, red onion, and parsley.

2. In a small bowl, whisk together the olive oil, lemon juice, salt, and pepper.

3. Pour the dressing over the turkey and avocado mixture and gently toss to coat everything evenly.

4. Serve the turkey and avocado salad chilled or at room temperature. It can be served on its own, on a bed of greens, or with whole grain crackers or bread.

This salad is a great option for those with diabetes or high cholesterol for a few reasons:

- Turkey is a lean protein that is low in saturated fat and high in protein.

- Avocado provides healthy monounsaturated fats that can help lower cholesterol.

- The salad is low in carbs and high in fiber, vitamins, and minerals.

- The olive oil and lemon juice dressing is a healthier alternative to creamy dressings.

This makes for a nutritious, filling, and delicious meal or snack. Enjoy!

61. Baked tilapia with lemon and garlic

Ingredient:

- 4 tilapia fillets (about 1 lb total)
- 2 tablespoons olive oil
- 3 cloves garlic, minced
- 1 tablespoon lemon juice
- 1 teaspoon lemon zest
- 1/2 teaspoon dried parsley
- 1/4 teaspoon salt
- 1/4 teaspoon black pepper

Instructions:

1. Preheat your oven to 400°F. Lightly grease a baking dish or line a baking sheet with parchment paper.

2. In a small bowl, mix together the olive oil, minced garlic, lemon juice, lemon zest, dried parsley, salt, and pepper.

3. Place the tilapia fillets in the prepared baking dish or on the baking sheet. Spoon the lemon•garlic mixture evenly over the top of the fish, making sure to coat all the fillets.

4. Bake the tilapia for 15•18 minutes, or until it flakes easily with a fork and reaches an internal temperature of 145°F.

5. Serve the baked tilapia with lemon and garlic warm, garnished with additional lemon wedges if desired.

Tips:
- You can use any white fish fillets, such as cod or halibut, in place of the tilapia.

- For extra flavor, you can add a sprinkle of Parmesan cheese or chopped fresh herbs on top before baking.

- Serve the baked tilapia with roasted vegetables, a fresh salad, or steamed rice for a complete and healthy meal.

This baked tilapia with lemon and garlic is a simple, yet flavorful dish that's perfect for a quick weeknight dinner. The bright, garlicky flavors complement the mild, flaky fish perfectly. Enjoy!

62. Grilled chicken with mango salsa

Ingredient:

Mango Salsa:
- 1 ripe mango, diced
- 1/2 red onion, finely chopped
- 1 jalapeño, seeded and finely chopped
- 1/4 cup chopped fresh cilantro
- 2 tbsp lime juice
- 1/4 tsp salt

Grilled Chicken:
- 4 boneless, skinless chicken breasts
- 1 tbsp olive oil
- 1 tsp chili powder
- 1/2 tsp garlic powder
- 1/4 tsp salt
- 1/4 tsp black pepper

Instructions:

1. Make the mango salsa: In a medium bowl, combine the diced mango, red onion, jalapeño, cilantro, lime juice, and 1/4 tsp salt. Stir to mix well and set aside.

2. Prepare the chicken: Preheat grill or grill pan to medium•high heat.

3. Rub the chicken breasts all over with the olive oil, chili powder, garlic powder, salt, and pepper.

4. Grill the chicken for 5•7 minutes per side, until cooked through and no longer pink in the center.

5. Serve the grilled chicken topped with the fresh mango salsa.

This dish is a great option for those with diabetes or high cholesterol for a few reasons:

- Chicken is a lean protein that is low in saturated fat.
- Mangoes are a good source of fiber, vitamins, and antioxidants.
- The salsa is low in calories and added sugars.
- Olive oil provides healthy monounsaturated fats.
- The dish is low in sodium and carbs.

The sweet and spicy mango salsa pairs perfectly with the grilled chicken for a flavorful and nutritious meal. Enjoy!

63. Tofu and vegetable stir•fry

Ingredient:

- 1 block (14 oz) extra•firm tofu, cubed
- 2 tbsp sesame oil, divided
- 2 cups mixed vegetables (such as broccoli, bell peppers, snap peas, carrots)
- 3 cloves garlic, minced
- 1 tbsp grated fresh ginger
- 2 tbsp low•sodium soy sauce or tamari
- 1 tsp rice vinegar
- 1 tsp honey (optional)
- Salt and pepper to taste
- Chopped green onions for garnish (optional)

Instructions:

1. Pat the tofu cubes dry with paper towels to remove excess moisture.

2. In a large skillet or wok, heat 1 tbsp of the sesame oil over medium•high heat. Add the tofu cubes and cook for 5•7 minutes, turning occasionally, until lightly browned on all sides. Transfer the tofu to a plate.

3. Add the remaining 1 tbsp of sesame oil to the skillet. Add the mixed vegetables and stir•fry for 3•5 minutes until tender•crisp.

4. Add the garlic and ginger and cook for 1 minute, until fragrant.

5. Return the cooked tofu to the skillet. Pour in the soy sauce, rice vinegar, and honey (if using). Toss everything together and cook for 2•3 minutes until heated through.

6. Season with salt and pepper to taste.

7. Serve the tofu and vegetable stir•fry over steamed brown rice or quinoa. Garnish with chopped green onions if desired.

This stir•fry is a great option for those with diabetes or high cholesterol because:

- Tofu is a lean, plant•based protein that's low in saturated fat.
- The vegetables provide fiber, vitamins, and minerals.
- The dish is low in sodium and added sugars.
- The sesame oil and soy sauce provide flavor without the need for heavy sauces.

64. Zucchini noodles with tomato sauce

Ingredient:

- 3 medium zucchinis, spiralized or julienned into noodles
- 1 tbsp olive oil
- 1/2 onion, diced
- 3 cloves garlic, minced
- 1 (14 oz) can diced tomatoes
- 2 tbsp tomato paste
- 1 tsp dried oregano
- 1/4 tsp red pepper flakes (optional)
- Salt and pepper to taste
- Grated Parmesan cheese (optional)

Instructions:

1. Using a spiralizer or julienne peeler, cut the zucchinis into long, thin noodles. Set aside.

2. In a large skillet, heat the olive oil over medium heat. Add the onion and sauté for 3•4 minutes until translucent.

3. Add the garlic and cook for 1 minute, until fragrant.

4. Stir in the diced tomatoes, tomato paste, oregano, and red pepper flakes (if using). Bring the sauce to a simmer and let it cook for 5•7 minutes, until slightly thickened.

5. Add the zucchini noodles to the sauce and toss to coat. Cook for 2•3 minutes, just until the zucchini is tender but still crisp.

6. Season with salt and pepper to taste.

7. Serve the zucchini noodles with the tomato sauce, topped with a sprinkle of Parmesan cheese if desired.

This dish is a great option for those with diabetes or high cholesterol for a few reasons:

- Zucchini noodles are low in carbs and calories, making them a healthier alternative to pasta.
- The tomato sauce is low in sodium and added sugars.
- The olive oil provides heart•healthy monounsaturated fats.
- The dish is high in fiber, vitamins, and antioxidants from the vegetables.

65. Cauliflower rice with stir•fried vegetables

Ingredient:

• 1 head of cauliflower, cut into florets
• 1 tbsp olive oil
• 1 cup sliced mushrooms
• 1 cup sliced bell peppers
• 1 cup broccoli florets
• 1 cup snow peas or snap peas
• 2 cloves garlic, minced
• 1 tsp grated ginger
• 2 tbsp low•sodium soy sauce or tamari
• 1 tsp sesame oil
• Salt and pepper to taste
• Chopped green onions for garnish (optional)

Instructions:

1. In a food processor, pulse the cauliflower florets until they resemble rice•sized grains. Set aside.

2. In a large skillet or wok, heat the olive oil over medium•high heat.

3. Add the mushrooms, bell peppers, broccoli, and snow/snap peas. Stir•fry for 5•7 minutes until the vegetables are tender•crisp.

4. Add the garlic and ginger and cook for 1 minute, until fragrant.

5. Stir in the cauliflower rice, soy sauce, and sesame oil. Cook for 3•5 minutes, stirring frequently, until the cauliflower rice is heated through.

6. Season with salt and pepper to taste. Serve the cauliflower rice and stir•fried vegetables warm, garnished with chopped green onions if desired.

This dish is a great option for those with diabetes or high cholesterol for a few reasons:

• Cauliflower rice is low in carbs and calories, making it a healthier alternative to regular rice.
• The stir•fried vegetables provide fiber, vitamins, and minerals.
• The dish is low in sodium and contains healthy fats from the olive and sesame oils.
• It's a filling and satisfying meal that's easy to prepare.

66. Greek salad with grilled shrimp

Ingredient:

Salad:
- 5 oz mixed greens
- 1 cup cherry tomatoes, halved
- 1/2 cucumber, sliced
- 1/4 red onion, thinly sliced
- 1/2 cup crumbled feta cheese
- 1/4 cup kalamata olives, pitted and halved

Dressing:
- 2 tbsp olive oil
- 1 tbsp red wine vinegar
- 1 tsp Dijon mustard
- 1 tsp dried oregano
- 1 clove garlic, minced
- Salt and pepper to taste

Shrimp:
- 1 lb large shrimp, peeled and deveined
- 1 tbsp olive oil
- 1 tsp dried oregano
- 1/4 tsp salt
- 1/4 tsp black pepper

Instructions:

1. Preheat grill or grill pan to medium•high heat.

2. In a medium bowl, toss the shrimp with the 1 tbsp olive oil, 1 tsp oregano, salt, and pepper.

3. Grill the shrimp for 2•3 minutes per side, until opaque and cooked through. Set aside.

4. In a large salad bowl, combine the mixed greens, tomatoes, cucumber, red onion, feta, and olives.

5. In a small bowl, whisk together the dressing ingredients • 2 tbsp olive oil, vinegar, mustard, 1 tsp oregano, garlic, salt and pepper.

6. Add the grilled shrimp to the salad and drizzle the dressing over top. Toss gently to coat. Serve the Greek salad with grilled shrimp immediately.

This salad is a great option for those with diabetes or high cholesterol for a few reasons:

- Shrimp is a lean protein that is low in saturated fat. The salad is loaded with fiber•rich vegetables.
- The dressing uses heart•healthy olive oil and minimal added sugars.
- The feta cheese provides calcium and protein. The overall dish is low in carbs and calories.

67. Tuna and avocado wrap

Ingredient:

- 1 (5 oz) can tuna, drained and flaked
- 1/2 avocado, diced
- 2 tbsp plain Greek yogurt
- 1 tsp lemon juice
- 1/4 tsp dried dill
- Salt and pepper to taste
- 2 whole wheat tortillas or wraps

Instructions:

1. In a medium bowl, combine the tuna, avocado, Greek yogurt, lemon juice, and dried dill. Mix well and season with salt and pepper to taste.

2. Lay the tortillas or wraps out flat. Divide the tuna and avocado mixture evenly between the two wraps, spreading it in a line down the center.

3. Fold the bottom of the wrap up over the filling, then fold in the sides and continue rolling up tightly to enclose the filling.

4. Slice the wraps in half diagonally and serve.

This tuna and avocado wrap is a great option for those with diabetes or high cholesterol for a few reasons:

- Tuna is a lean protein that is low in saturated fat and high in omega•3 fatty acids.

- Avocado provides heart•healthy monounsaturated fats.

- Greek yogurt adds protein and creaminess without a lot of fat or calories.

- Whole wheat tortillas are a good source of complex carbs and fiber.

- The dish is low in sodium and added sugars.

This wrap makes for a filling and nutritious lunch or snack. The combination of tuna, avocado, and the creamy yogurt dressing is both delicious and good for you. Enjoy!

68. Roasted Brussels sprouts with cranberries

Ingredient:

- 1 lb Brussels sprouts, trimmed and halved
- 2 tbsp olive oil
- 1/4 tsp salt
- 1/4 tsp black pepper
- 1/2 cup fresh or frozen cranberries
- 1 tbsp honey (optional)

Instructions:

1. Preheat oven to 400°F. Line a baking sheet with parchment paper.

2. In a large bowl, toss the Brussels sprouts with the olive oil, salt, and pepper until evenly coated.

3. Spread the Brussels sprouts in a single layer on the prepared baking sheet.

4. Roast for 15 minutes, then add the cranberries to the pan and continue roasting for 10•15 minutes more, until the Brussels sprouts are tender and lightly browned.

5. If desired, drizzle the roasted Brussels sprouts and cranberries with the honey and toss to coat.

6. Serve warm.

This dish is a great option for those with diabetes or high cholesterol for a few reasons:

- Brussels sprouts are high in fiber, vitamins, and minerals, and low in carbs.

- Cranberries are a source of antioxidants and can help support heart health.

- The olive oil provides healthy monounsaturated fats.

- The honey is optional, so you can control the amount of added sugar.

The combination of the roasted Brussels sprouts and tart cranberries makes for a delicious and nutritious side dish. Enjoy!

69. Baked salmon with garlic butter

Ingredient:

- 4 (6 oz) salmon fillets
- 2 tbsp unsalted butter, softened
- 2 cloves garlic, minced
- 1 tbsp chopped fresh parsley
- 1/4 tsp salt
- 1/4 tsp black pepper

Instructions:

1. Preheat oven to 400°F. Line a baking sheet with parchment paper.

2. In a small bowl, mix together the softened butter, garlic, parsley, salt and pepper until well combined.

3. Place the salmon fillets on the prepared baking sheet. Spread the garlic butter evenly over the top of each fillet.

4. Bake for 12•15 minutes, until the salmon is opaque and flakes easily with a fork.

5. Serve the baked salmon immediately, garnished with extra parsley if desired.

This recipe is perfect for those with diabetes and high cholesterol for a few reasons:

- Salmon is an excellent source of heart•healthy omega•3 fatty acids, which can help lower triglycerides and cholesterol levels.

- The garlic butter adds flavor without the need for high•sodium sauces or marinades.

- Baking the salmon is a healthier cooking method compared to frying.

- The portion size of 6 oz of salmon per serving is appropriate for a diabetic•friendly meal.

Enjoy this delicious and nutritious baked salmon dish!

70. Shrimp and quinoa salad

Ingredient:

- 1 cup cooked quinoa, cooled
- 1 lb cooked shrimp, peeled and deveined
- 1 cup cherry tomatoes, halved
- 1 cucumber, diced
- 1/2 cup crumbled feta cheese
- 1/4 cup chopped fresh parsley
- 2 tbsp olive oil
- 2 tbsp lemon juice
- 1 tsp Dijon mustard
- 1/4 tsp salt
- 1/4 tsp black pepper

Instructions:

1. In a large bowl, combine the cooked quinoa, shrimp, tomatoes, cucumber, feta and parsley.

2. In a small bowl, whisk together the olive oil, lemon juice, Dijon mustard, salt and pepper.

3. Pour the dressing over the quinoa salad and toss gently to coat.

4. Serve chilled or at room temperature.

This shrimp and quinoa salad is a great option for those with diabetes and high cholesterol for a few reasons:

- Quinoa is a high•fiber, high•protein grain that is low in carbs, making it diabetes•friendly.

- Shrimp is a lean protein that is low in saturated fat and cholesterol.

- The olive oil•based dressing is heart•healthy compared to creamy dressings.

- The fresh vegetables and herbs provide antioxidants and nutrients.

- The portion size is balanced and appropriate for a main dish salad.

This salad is refreshing, flavorful and nutritious. Enjoy!

71. Eggplant lasagna

Ingredient:

- 1/4 tsp red pepper flakes (optional)
- Salt and pepper to taste
- 1 cup part•skim ricotta cheese
- 1 egg
- 1/4 cup grated Parmesan cheese
- 2 cups shredded part•skim mozzarella cheese

- 2 medium eggplants, sliced lengthwise into 1/4•inch thick slices
- 2 tbsp olive oil
- 1 onion, diced
- 3 cloves garlic, minced
- 1 (28 oz) can crushed tomatoes
- 2 tsp dried oregano

Instructions:

1. Preheat oven to 375°F. Lightly grease a 9x13 inch baking dish.

2. Arrange the eggplant slices in a single layer on a baking sheet. Brush both sides with olive oil. Roast for 15•20 minutes, flipping halfway, until tender.

3. In a large skillet, heat 1 tbsp olive oil over medium heat. Add the onion and sauté for 5 minutes until translucent. Add the garlic and cook for 1 minute more.

4. Stir in the crushed tomatoes, oregano, red pepper flakes (if using), and season with salt and pepper. Simmer for 10 minutes.

5. In a small bowl, mix together the ricotta, egg, and Parmesan.

6. Spread 1 cup of the tomato sauce in the bottom of the prepared baking dish. Layer half of the roasted eggplant slices over the sauce. Spread the ricotta mixture over the eggplant, then top with 1 cup of the mozzarella.

7. Add another layer of eggplant, then the remaining tomato sauce. Top with the remaining mozzarella cheese.

8. Bake for 30•35 minutes, until the cheese is melted and bubbly. Let stand for 10 minutes before serving.

This eggplant lasagna is a great option for those with diabetes or high cholesterol because:

- Eggplant is low in carbs and calories, making it a healthier alternative to traditional pasta.
- The dish is high in fiber, vitamins, and antioxidants from the vegetables.
- It uses part•skim cheeses to reduce saturated fat. There are no added sugars.

72. Spinach and goat cheese stuffed turkey meatballs

Ingredient:

- 1 lb ground turkey
- 1 cup fresh spinach, finely chopped
- 2 oz crumbled goat cheese
- 1/4 cup whole wheat breadcrumbs
- 1 egg, lightly beaten
- 2 tbsp minced onion
- 2 cloves garlic, minced
- 1 tsp dried oregano
- 1/4 tsp salt
- 1/4 tsp black pepper

Instructions:

1. Preheat oven to 400°F. Line a baking sheet with parchment paper.

2. In a large bowl, combine the ground turkey, spinach, goat cheese, breadcrumbs, egg, onion, garlic, oregano, salt and pepper. Mix well until fully incorporated.

3. Scoop out about 2 tablespoons of the mixture and roll into a ball. Place on the prepared baking sheet. Repeat with remaining mixture.

4. Bake for 18•20 minutes, until meatballs are cooked through and no longer pink in the center.

5. Serve warm. Enjoy!

These meatballs are a great source of lean protein from the turkey, while the spinach and goat cheese provide nutrients and flavor. The whole wheat breadcrumbs help keep them diabetes•friendly. Enjoy!

73. Chickpea and spinach curry

Ingredient:

- 1 tbsp olive oil
- 1 onion, diced
- 3 cloves garlic, minced
- 1 tbsp grated fresh ginger
- 1 tsp ground cumin
- 1 tsp ground coriander
- 1 tsp garam masala
- 1/4 tsp cayenne pepper (optional)
- 1 (15 oz) can chickpeas, rinsed and drained
- 1 (14 oz) can diced tomatoes
- 1 cup low•sodium vegetable broth
- 4 cups fresh spinach, chopped
- 1/4 cup plain Greek yogurt (optional)
- Salt and pepper to taste

Instructions:

1. In a large skillet or pot, heat the olive oil over medium heat. Add the onion and sauté for 5 minutes until translucent.

2. Add the garlic, ginger, cumin, coriander, garam masala, and cayenne (if using). Cook for 1 minute, stirring constantly, until fragrant.

3. Stir in the chickpeas, diced tomatoes, and vegetable broth. Bring to a simmer and cook for 10•15 minutes, until slightly thickened.

4. Add the chopped spinach and cook for 2•3 minutes until wilted.

5. Remove from heat and stir in the Greek yogurt, if using. Season with salt and pepper to taste. Serve the chickpea and spinach curry over basmati rice or with naan bread.

This curry is a great option for those with diabetes or high cholesterol because:

- Chickpeas are a good source of plant•based protein and fiber.

- Spinach is packed with vitamins, minerals, and antioxidants.

- The spices provide flavor without added salt or sugar.

- The Greek yogurt adds a creamy texture and protein.

74. Turkey and quinoa stuffed zucchini

Ingredient:

- 4 medium zucchini, halved lengthwise
- 1 lb ground turkey
- 1 cup cooked quinoa
- 1/2 cup diced onion

- 2 cloves garlic, minced
- 1 tsp dried oregano
- 1/4 tsp salt
- 1/4 tsp black pepper
- 1 cup marinara sauce
- 1/2 cup shredded part•skim mozzarella cheese

Instructions:

1. Preheat oven to 375°F. Spray a baking dish with non•stick cooking spray.

2. Scoop out the flesh from the zucchini halves, leaving about 1/4 inch of the zucchini shell. Finely chop the scooped out zucchini flesh.

3. In a skillet over medium heat, cook the ground turkey, chopped zucchini flesh, onion and garlic until the turkey is browned and the vegetables are tender, about 5•7 minutes. Drain any excess fat.

4. Stir in the cooked quinoa, oregano, salt and pepper.

5. Spoon the turkey•quinoa mixture into the zucchini shells, packing it in tightly.

6. Place the stuffed zucchini halves in the prepared baking dish. Top each one with 2•3 tablespoons of marinara sauce and sprinkle with the mozzarella cheese.

7. Bake for 20•25 minutes, until the zucchini is tender and the cheese is melted. Serve hot.

This turkey and quinoa stuffed zucchini dish is a great option for those with diabetes and high cholesterol for a few reasons:

- Zucchini is a low•carb, high•fiber vegetable that is diabetes•friendly.
- Ground turkey is a lean protein that is low in saturated fat and cholesterol.
- Quinoa is a high•protein, high•fiber grain that helps keep blood sugar stable.
- The marinara sauce provides lycopene and other antioxidants.
- The use of part•skim mozzarella keeps the saturated fat and cholesterol content low.
- Baking instead of frying is a healthier cooking method.
- The portion size is balanced and appropriate for a main dish.

75. Baked eggplant with mozzarella

Ingredient:

- 1 medium eggplant, sliced into 1/2•inch rounds
- 1 tbsp olive oil
- 1/4 tsp salt
- 1/4 tsp black pepper
- 1 cup marinara sauce
- 1 cup shredded part•skim mozzarella cheese
- 2 tbsp grated Parmesan cheese
- 2 tbsp chopped fresh basil

Instructions:

1. Preheat oven to 400°F. Line a baking sheet with parchment paper.

2. Arrange the eggplant slices in a single layer on the prepared baking sheet. Brush the tops with olive oil and season with salt and pepper.

3. Bake for 15•20 minutes, flipping halfway, until the eggplant is tender.

4. Remove the eggplant from the oven and top each slice with a spoonful of marinara sauce, followed by the mozzarella and Parmesan cheeses.

5. Return the baking sheet to the oven and bake for an additional 5•7 minutes, until the cheese is melted and bubbly.

6. Garnish the baked eggplant with the chopped fresh basil before serving.

This baked eggplant dish is a great option for those with diabetes and high cholesterol for a few reasons:

- Eggplant is a low•carb, high•fiber vegetable that is diabetes•friendly.
- The use of part•skim mozzarella and a small amount of Parmesan keeps the saturated fat and cholesterol content low.
- Baking instead of frying the eggplant is a healthier cooking method.
- The marinara sauce provides lycopene and other antioxidants.
- The portion size is balanced and appropriate for a main dish.

Enjoy this delicious and nutritious baked eggplant recipe!

76. Grilled shrimp with cilantro lime sauce

Ingredient:

- 1 lb large shrimp, peeled and deveined
- 2 tbsp olive oil
- 1 tsp chili powder
- 1/4 tsp salt
- 1/4 tsp black pepper

Cilantro Lime Sauce:
- 1/4 cup plain Greek yogurt
- 2 tbsp chopped fresh cilantro
- 1 tbsp lime juice
- 1 clove garlic, minced
- 1/4 tsp salt
- 1/4 tsp black pepper

Instructions:

1. In a large bowl, toss the shrimp with the olive oil, chili powder, salt and pepper until evenly coated.

2. Preheat grill or grill pan to medium•high heat.

3. Grill the shrimp for 2•3 minutes per side, until opaque and cooked through.

4. In a small bowl, mix together the Greek yogurt, cilantro, lime juice, garlic, salt and pepper for the cilantro lime sauce.

5. Serve the grilled shrimp warm, drizzled with the cilantro lime sauce.

This grilled shrimp dish is a great option for those with diabetes and high cholesterol for a few reasons:

- Shrimp is a lean protein that is low in saturated fat and cholesterol.
- The cilantro lime sauce is made with Greek yogurt, which provides protein and probiotics.
- Grilling the shrimp is a healthy cooking method that doesn't require added oils or butter.
- The portion size of 1 lb of shrimp is appropriate for a main dish.
- The dish is low in carbs and high in protein, making it diabetes•friendly.

77. Cauliflower crust pizza with mushrooms and olives

Ingredient:

- 1 head cauliflower, riced (about 3 cups riced)
- 1 egg, lightly beaten
- 1/2 cup shredded part•skim mozzarella cheese
- 2 tbsp grated Parmesan cheese
- 1/4 tsp garlic powder
- 1/4 tsp dried oregano
- 1/4 tsp salt

Topping Ingredients:
- 1/2 cup marinara sauce
- 1 cup sliced mushrooms
- 1/4 cup sliced black olives
- 1/2 cup shredded part•skim mozzarella cheese

Instructions:

1. Preheat oven to 400°F. Line a baking sheet with parchment paper.

2. Make the cauliflower crust: In a food processor, pulse the cauliflower florets until they resemble rice. Transfer to a clean kitchen towel and squeeze out as much moisture as possible.

3. In a bowl, mix the riced cauliflower, egg, mozzarella, Parmesan, garlic powder, oregano and salt until well combined.

4. Press the cauliflower mixture onto the prepared baking sheet, forming a thin round crust. Bake for 20•25 minutes until golden brown.

5. Top the baked crust with the marinara sauce, mushrooms, olives and mozzarella cheese.

6. Return the pizza to the oven and bake for an additional 10•12 minutes, until the cheese is melted and bubbly. Slice and serve hot.

This cauliflower crust pizza is a great option for those with diabetes and high cholesterol for a few reasons:

- The cauliflower crust is low in carbs and high in fiber, making it diabetes•friendly.
- The use of part•skim mozzarella and a small amount of Parmesan keeps the saturated fat and cholesterol content low.
- Mushrooms and olives are nutrient•dense toppings that provide antioxidants.
- Baking the pizza is a healthier cooking method compared to traditional pizza.
- The portion size is balanced and appropriate for a main dish.

78. Greek yogurt with honey and berries

Ingredient:

- 1 cup plain, unsweetened Greek yogurt
- 1 tbsp raw honey
- 1/2 cup mixed fresh berries (such as blueberries, raspberries, strawberries)
- 1 tbsp chopped walnuts (optional)

Instructions:

1. In a bowl, spoon the Greek yogurt and drizzle the honey over the top.

2. Gently fold the honey into the yogurt until well combined.

3. Top the honey•sweetened yogurt with the mixed fresh berries.

4. If desired, sprinkle the chopped walnuts over the top.

This Greek yogurt parfait is a great option for those with diabetes and high cholesterol for a few reasons:

- Greek yogurt is high in protein and low in carbs, making it a diabetes•friendly choice.

- The natural sweetness from the honey provides a touch of sweetness without spiking blood sugar levels.

- Berries are low in carbs and high in fiber, vitamins, and antioxidants.

- Walnuts are a source of heart•healthy omega•3 fatty acids.

- The portion size is balanced and appropriate for a healthy snack or light meal.

This simple yet delicious parfait is a nutritious way to satisfy your sweet tooth while supporting your health goals. Enjoy!

79. Baked chicken with sun•dried tomatoes

Ingredient:

- 4 boneless, skinless chicken breasts
- 1/4 cup chopped sun•dried tomatoes (not oil•packed)
- 2 tbsp chopped fresh basil
- 2 cloves garlic, minced
- 1 tbsp olive oil
- 1/4 tsp salt
- 1/4 tsp black pepper

Instructions:

1. Preheat oven to 400°F. Lightly grease a baking dish.

2. In a small bowl, combine the sun•dried tomatoes, basil, garlic, olive oil, salt and pepper.

3. Place the chicken breasts in the prepared baking dish. Spoon the sun•dried tomato mixture evenly over the top of the chicken.

4. Bake for 25•30 minutes, until the chicken is cooked through and reaches an internal temperature of 165°F.

5. Serve the baked chicken immediately, spooning any extra sauce from the baking dish over the top.

This baked chicken dish is a great option for those with diabetes and high cholesterol for a few reasons:

- Chicken breast is a lean protein that is low in saturated fat and cholesterol.

- Sun•dried tomatoes are a good source of lycopene, an antioxidant that may help lower cholesterol.

- Fresh basil adds flavor without the need for high•sodium seasonings.

- Baking the chicken is a healthier cooking method compared to frying.

- The portion size of 1 chicken breast is appropriate for a diabetic•friendly meal.

80. Lentil and kale soup

Ingredient:

- 1 tbsp olive oil
- 1 onion, diced
- 3 cloves garlic, minced
- 1 cup brown or green lentils, rinsed
- 6 cups low•sodium vegetable or chicken broth
- 1 (14 oz) can diced tomatoes
- 1 tsp dried thyme
- 1 tsp dried oregano
- 1/4 tsp red pepper flakes (optional)
- Salt and pepper to taste
- 4 cups chopped kale, stems removed

Instructions:

1. In a large pot or Dutch oven, heat the olive oil over medium heat. Add the onion and sauté for 5 minutes until translucent.

2. Add the garlic and cook for 1 minute, until fragrant.

3. Stir in the lentils, broth, diced tomatoes, thyme, oregano, and red pepper flakes (if using). Season with salt and pepper.

4. Bring the soup to a boil, then reduce heat and let it simmer for 20•25 minutes, until the lentils are tender.

5. Add the chopped kale and continue simmering for 5•10 minutes more, until the kale is wilted and tender. Taste and adjust seasonings as needed. Serve the lentil and kale soup hot.

This soup is a great option for those with diabetes or high cholesterol for a few reasons:

- Lentils are an excellent source of plant•based protein and fiber, which can help regulate blood sugar levels.

- Kale is packed with vitamins, minerals, and antioxidants, and is low in calories.

- The soup is low in sodium and contains no added sugars. The olive oil provides heart•healthy monounsaturated fats.

81. Turkey and vegetable stir•fry with quinoa

Ingredient:

- 1 cup cooked quinoa
- 1 lb ground turkey
- 2 tbsp low•sodium soy sauce
- 1 tsp sesame oil
- 1 tsp grated fresh ginger
- 2 cloves garlic, minced
- 1 cup broccoli florets
- 1 cup sliced mushrooms

- 1 cup sliced bell peppers
- 1/2 cup sliced snow peas
- 2 tbsp chopped green onions
- 1 tbsp sesame seeds (optional)

Sauce:

- 2 tbsp low•sodium soy sauce
- 1 tbsp rice vinegar
- 1 tsp honey
- 1/4 tsp red pepper flakes (optional)

Instructions:

1. Cook the quinoa according to package instructions. Set aside.

2. In a large skillet or wok, cook the ground turkey over medium•high heat, breaking it up as it cooks, until no longer pink, about 5•7 minutes. Drain any excess fat.

3. Add the 2 tbsp soy sauce, sesame oil, ginger and garlic to the turkey. Stir and cook for 1 minute.

4. Add the broccoli, mushrooms, bell peppers and snow peas. Stir•fry for 3•5 minutes until the vegetables are tender•crisp.

5. In a small bowl, whisk together the sauce ingredients.

6. Add the cooked quinoa and sauce to the turkey and vegetable mixture. Toss to combine and heat through, about 2 minutes. Garnish with the chopped green onions and sesame seeds (if using) before serving.

This turkey and vegetable stir•fry with quinoa is a great option for those with diabetes and high cholesterol for a few reasons:

- Ground turkey is a lean protein that is low in saturated fat and cholesterol.
- Quinoa is a high•fiber, high•protein grain that helps keep blood sugar stable.
- The vegetables provide fiber, vitamins, minerals and antioxidants.
- The sauce is made with low•sodium soy sauce, rice vinegar and a touch of honey for flavor.
- Stir•frying is a quick, healthy cooking method that doesn't require added oils or butter.
- The portion size is balanced and appropriate for a diabetic•friendly main dish.

82. Baked trout with almond butter sauce

Ingredient:

- 4 (6 oz) trout fillets
- 1 tbsp olive oil
- 1/4 tsp salt
- 1/4 tsp black pepper

Almond Butter Sauce:
- 2 tbsp unsalted almond butter
- 2 tbsp low•sodium chicken or vegetable broth
- 1 tbsp lemon juice
- 1 tsp Dijon mustard
- 1 tsp honey
- 1/4 tsp garlic powder
- 1/4 tsp salt
- 1/4 tsp black pepper

Instructions:

1. Preheat oven to 400°F. Line a baking sheet with parchment paper.

2. Place the trout fillets on the prepared baking sheet. Brush the tops with the olive oil and season with salt and pepper.

3. Bake for 12•15 minutes, until the trout is opaque and flakes easily with a fork.

4. While the trout is baking, make the almond butter sauce. In a small bowl, whisk together all the sauce ingredients until smooth and well combined. Serve the baked trout fillets warm, drizzled with the almond butter sauce.

This baked trout with almond butter sauce is a great option for those with diabetes and high cholesterol for a few reasons:

- Trout is an excellent source of heart•healthy omega•3 fatty acids, which can help lower triglycerides and cholesterol levels.
- Almond butter provides healthy monounsaturated fats and is low in carbs, making it diabetes•friendly.
- The sauce is made with low•sodium broth, lemon juice, Dijon and honey, providing flavor without the need for high•sodium ingredients.
- Baking the trout is a healthier cooking method compared to frying.
- The portion size of 6 oz of trout per serving is appropriate for a diabetic•friendly meal.

83. Spinach and feta stuffed turkey breast

Ingredient:

- 1 lb boneless, skinless turkey breast
- 1 cup fresh spinach, chopped
- 1/2 cup crumbled feta cheese
- 2 tbsp chopped fresh dill
- 1 clove garlic, minced
- 1/4 tsp salt
- 1/4 tsp black pepper

Instructions:

1. Preheat oven to 375°F. Lightly grease a baking dish.

2. Slice the turkey breast horizontally to create a pocket, being careful not to cut all the way through.

3. In a bowl, mix together the spinach, feta, dill, garlic, salt and pepper until well combined.

4. Stuff the spinach•feta mixture into the pocket of the turkey breast.

5. Place the stuffed turkey breast in the prepared baking dish.

6. Bake for 30•35 minutes, until the turkey is cooked through and reaches an internal temperature of 165°F. Let the turkey rest for 5 minutes before slicing and serving.

This spinach and feta stuffed turkey breast is a great option for those with diabetes and high cholesterol for a few reasons:

- Turkey breast is a lean protein that is low in saturated fat and cholesterol.
- Spinach is a nutrient•dense vegetable that is low in carbs and high in fiber.
- Feta cheese is a lower•fat cheese option compared to other cheeses.
- The simple seasoning of dill, garlic, salt and pepper adds flavor without the need for high•sodium sauces or marinades.
- Baking the turkey is a healthier cooking method compared to frying.
- The portion size of 4•6 oz of turkey per serving is appropriate for a diabetic•friendly meal.

Serve this stuffed turkey breast with a side of roasted vegetables or a fresh salad for a complete, diabetes•friendly and heart•healthy meal. Enjoy!

84. Quinoa and black bean salad with avocado

Ingredient:

- 1 cup cooked quinoa, cooled
- 1 (15 oz) can black beans, rinsed and drained
- 1 cup diced cucumber
- 1/2 cup diced tomatoes
- 1/4 cup diced red onion
- 1 avocado, diced
- 2 tbsp chopped fresh cilantro
- 2 tbsp lime juice
- 1 tbsp olive oil
- 1/4 tsp salt
- 1/4 tsp black pepper

Instructions:

1. In a large bowl, combine the cooked quinoa, black beans, cucumber, tomatoes, red onion, avocado and cilantro.

2. In a small bowl, whisk together the lime juice, olive oil, salt and pepper to make the dressing.

3. Pour the dressing over the quinoa and bean salad and toss gently to coat.

4. Serve the quinoa and black bean salad chilled or at room temperature.

This quinoa and black bean salad is a great option for those with diabetes and high cholesterol for a few reasons:

- Quinoa is a high•fiber, high•protein grain that helps keep blood sugar stable.
- Black beans are a good source of fiber, protein and complex carbs, making them diabetes•friendly.
- Avocado provides heart•healthy monounsaturated fats that can help lower cholesterol.
- The fresh vegetables and herbs provide antioxidants and nutrients.
- The simple lime•olive oil dressing is low in sodium and calories.
- The portion size is balanced and appropriate for a main dish salad.

This salad is refreshing, flavorful and nutritious. Enjoy it as a light lunch or pair it with grilled chicken or fish for a complete, diabetes•friendly and heart•healthy meal.

85. Turkey and vegetable kebabs with tzatziki sauce

Ingredient:

- 1 lb ground turkey
- 1 zucchini, cut into 1•inch pieces
- 1 red bell pepper, cut into 1•inch pieces
- 1 red onion, cut into 1•inch pieces
- 8 cherry tomatoes
- 1 tbsp olive oil
- 1/2 tsp dried oregano
- 1/4 tsp salt
- 1/4 tsp black pepper

Tzatziki Sauce:
- 1 cup plain Greek yogurt
- 1/2 cucumber, peeled, seeded and grated
- 1 clove garlic, minced
- 1 tbsp chopped fresh dill
- 1 tbsp lemon juice
- 1/4 tsp salt
- 1/4 tsp black pepper

Instructions:

1. Preheat grill or grill pan to medium•high heat.

2. In a bowl, gently mix together the ground turkey, zucchini, bell pepper, onion, tomatoes, olive oil, oregano, salt and pepper until well combined.

3. Thread the turkey and vegetable pieces onto skewers, alternating the ingredients.

4. Grill the kebabs for 12•15 minutes, turning occasionally, until the turkey is cooked through and the vegetables are tender.

5. In a small bowl, mix together all the tzatziki sauce ingredients until well combined.

6. Serve the grilled turkey and vegetable kebabs warm, with the tzatziki sauce on the side for dipping.

This turkey and vegetable kebab dish is a great option for those with diabetes and high cholesterol for a few reasons:

- Ground turkey is a lean protein that is low in saturated fat and cholesterol.
- The vegetables provide fiber, vitamins, minerals and antioxidants.
- The tzatziki sauce is made with plain Greek yogurt, which is high in protein and probiotics.
- Grilling the kebabs is a healthy cooking method that doesn't require added oils or butter. The portion size is balanced and appropriate for a main dish.

Enjoy these flavorful and nutritious turkey and vegetable kebabs with the cool and creamy tzatziki sauce!

86. Baked sweet potato wedges

Ingredient:

- 2 medium sweet potatoes, scrubbed and cut into 1/2•inch thick wedges
- 1 tbsp olive oil
- 1/2 tsp paprika
- 1/4 tsp garlic powder
- 1/4 tsp salt
- 1/4 tsp black pepper

Instructions:

1. Preheat oven to 400°F. Line a baking sheet with parchment paper.

2. In a large bowl, toss the sweet potato wedges with the olive oil, paprika, garlic powder, salt and pepper until evenly coated.

3. Arrange the seasoned sweet potato wedges in a single layer on the prepared baking sheet.

4. Bake for 20•25 minutes, flipping halfway, until the wedges are tender and lightly browned.

5. Serve the baked sweet potato wedges hot.

This baked sweet potato recipe is a great option for those with diabetes and high cholesterol for a few reasons:

- Sweet potatoes are a complex carbohydrate that is high in fiber, vitamins, and minerals. They have a lower glycemic index compared to regular potatoes, making them a better choice for diabetics.
- Sweet potatoes are rich in beta•carotene, an antioxidant that may help lower cholesterol levels.
- Baking the sweet potato wedges instead of frying them keeps the fat and calorie content low.
- The simple seasoning of paprika, garlic, salt and pepper adds flavor without the need for high•sodium sauces or dressings.
- The portion size of 1•2 medium sweet potatoes per serving is appropriate for a diabetic•friendly side dish.

Enjoy these crispy, flavorful baked sweet potato wedges as a healthy alternative to traditional french fries or potato side dishes. They pair well with grilled or baked proteins for a complete, diabetes•friendly and heart•healthy meal.

87. Grilled chicken and vegetable skewers with balsamic glaze

Ingredient:

- 1 lb boneless, skinless chicken breasts, cut into 1•inch cubes
- 1 zucchini, cut into 1•inch pieces
- 1 red bell pepper, cut into 1•inch pieces
- 1 red onion, cut into 1•inch pieces
- 8 cherry tomatoes
- 2 tbsp olive oil
- 1/4 tsp salt
- 1/4 tsp black pepper

Balsamic Glaze:

- 1/4 cup balsamic vinegar
- 1 tbsp honey
- 1 tsp Dijon mustard
- 1/4 tsp salt

Instructions:

1. Preheat grill or grill pan to medium•high heat.

2. Thread the chicken, zucchini, bell pepper, onion and tomatoes onto skewers, alternating the ingredients.

3. Brush the skewers lightly with olive oil and season with salt and pepper.

4. Grill the skewers for 12•15 minutes, turning occasionally, until the chicken is cooked through and the vegetables are tender.

5. While the skewers are grilling, make the balsamic glaze. In a small saucepan, combine the balsamic vinegar, honey, Dijon and salt. Bring to a simmer and cook for 5•7 minutes, stirring occasionally, until thickened slightly. Serve the grilled chicken and vegetable skewers warm, drizzled with the balsamic glaze.

This grilled chicken and vegetable skewer dish is a great option for those with diabetes and high cholesterol for a few reasons:

- Chicken breast is a lean protein that is low in saturated fat and cholesterol.
- The vegetables provide fiber, vitamins, minerals and antioxidants.
- The balsamic glaze is made with a small amount of honey for sweetness, rather than sugar.
- Grilling the skewers is a healthy cooking method that doesn't require added oils or butter. The portion size is balanced and appropriate for a main dish.

Enjoy these flavorful and nutritious grilled chicken and vegetable skewers with the sweet and tangy balsamic glaze!

88. Tofu stir•fry with snow peas and carrots

Ingredient:

- 1 block (14 oz) extra•firm tofu, cubed
- 2 tbsp low•sodium soy sauce
- 1 tbsp rice vinegar
- 1 tsp sesame oil
- 1 tsp honey
- 1 tbsp olive oil
- 2 cloves garlic, minced
- 1 cup sliced snow peas
- 1 cup sliced carrots
- 1/2 cup sliced mushrooms
- 2 green onions, sliced
- 1 tsp sesame seeds (optional)

Instructions:

1. In a small bowl, whisk together the soy sauce, rice vinegar, sesame oil and honey. Set aside.

2. Heat the olive oil in a large skillet or wok over medium•high heat. Add the tofu cubes and cook for 3•4 minutes per side until lightly browned. Transfer the tofu to a plate.

3. Add the garlic, snow peas, carrots and mushrooms to the skillet. Stir•fry for 4•5 minutes until the vegetables are tender•crisp.

4. Return the tofu to the skillet and pour in the soy sauce mixture. Toss everything together and cook for 2•3 minutes until heated through.

5. Remove from heat and stir in the sliced green onions. Serve the tofu stir•fry hot, garnished with sesame seeds if desired. Enjoy!

This tofu stir•fry is a great option for those with diabetes and high cholesterol for a few reasons:

- Tofu is a plant•based protein that is low in saturated fat and cholesterol.
- The vegetables provide fiber, vitamins, minerals and antioxidants.
- The soy sauce, rice vinegar and honey provide flavor without the need for high•sodium ingredients.
- Stir•frying is a quick, healthy cooking method that doesn't require added oils or butter.
- The portion size is balanced and appropriate for a diabetic•friendly main dish.

89. Zucchini noodles with creamy pesto sauce

Ingredient:

• 3 medium zucchini, spiralized or julienned into noodles
• 1/2 cup fresh basil leaves
• 2 tbsp pine nuts
• 2 tbsp grated Parmesan cheese
• 1 clove garlic
• 2 tbsp olive oil
• 2 tbsp plain Greek yogurt
• 1 tbsp lemon juice
• 1/4 tsp salt
• 1/4 tsp black pepper

Instructions:

1. In a food processor or blender, combine the basil, pine nuts, Parmesan, garlic, olive oil, yogurt, lemon juice, salt and pepper. Blend until a smooth pesto sauce forms.

2. In a large skillet, cook the zucchini noodles over medium heat for 2•3 minutes, just until they start to soften slightly. Drain any excess moisture.

3. Add the pesto sauce to the zucchini noodles and toss to coat evenly. Serve the zucchini noodles with pesto warm.

This zucchini noodle dish is a great option for those with diabetes and high cholesterol for a few reasons:

• Zucchini noodles are a low•carb, high•fiber alternative to traditional pasta.

• The pesto sauce is made with heart•healthy olive oil and pine nuts instead of cream or cheese•based sauces.

• Greek yogurt adds creaminess while providing protein and probiotics.

• The small amount of Parmesan cheese keeps the saturated fat content low.

• The dish is naturally gluten•free and vegetarian.

• The portion size is balanced and appropriate for a diabetic•friendly main dish.

Enjoy this flavorful and nutritious zucchini noodle dish as a lighter alternative to pasta. It's a great way to get in extra vegetables while satisfying your pasta cravings.

90. Cauliflower rice with roasted vegetables

Ingredient:

- 1 head cauliflower, riced
- 1 cup cubed butternut squash
- 1 cup broccoli florets
- 1 cup diced zucchini
- 1 red bell pepper, diced
- 1 tbsp olive oil
- 1/4 tsp salt
- 1/4 tsp black pepper
- 2 tbsp chopped fresh parsley

Instructions:

1. Preheat oven to 400°F. Line a baking sheet with parchment paper.

2. In a large bowl, toss the butternut squash, broccoli, zucchini and bell pepper with the olive oil, salt and pepper until evenly coated.

3. Spread the vegetables in a single layer on the prepared baking sheet. Roast for 20•25 minutes, stirring halfway, until the vegetables are tender and lightly browned.

4. While the vegetables are roasting, place the riced cauliflower in a large skillet over medium heat. Cook for 5•7 minutes, stirring occasionally, until the cauliflower is tender.

5. Remove the roasted vegetables from the oven and add them to the cooked cauliflower rice. Toss to combine.

6. Stir in the chopped parsley just before serving.Serve the cauliflower rice and roasted vegetable mixture warm.

This cauliflower rice dish is a great option for those with diabetes and high cholesterol for a few reasons:

- Cauliflower rice is a low•carb, high•fiber alternative to traditional rice.
- The roasted vegetables provide fiber, vitamins, minerals and antioxidants.
- The dish is naturally gluten•free and vegan.
- Roasting the vegetables brings out their natural sweetness without the need for added sugars or sauces.
- The portion size is balanced and appropriate for a diabetic•friendly side dish or main meal

91. Greek salad with grilled salmon

Ingredient:

- 6 cups chopped romaine lettuce
- 1 cup cherry tomatoes, halved
- 1/2 cup diced cucumber
- 1/4 cup sliced red onion
- 1/4 cup pitted kalamata olives
- 2 tbsp crumbled feta cheese

Salmon Ingredients:

- 4 (6 oz) salmon fillets
- 1 tbsp olive oil
- 1 tsp dried oregano
- 1/4 tsp salt
- 1/4 tsp black pepper

Dressing:

- 2 tbsp olive oil
- 1 tbsp red wine vinegar
- 1 tbsp lemon juice
- 1 tsp Dijon mustard
- 1 tsp dried oregano
- 1/4 tsp salt
- 1/4 tsp black pepper

Instructions:

1. Preheat grill or grill pan to medium•high heat.

2. Brush the salmon fillets with olive oil and season with oregano, salt and pepper.

3. Grill the salmon for 4•5 minutes per side, until cooked through.

4. In a large bowl, combine the romaine, tomatoes, cucumber, onion and olives.

5. In a small bowl, whisk together the dressing ingredients.

6. Add the dressing to the salad and toss to coat.

7. Divide the salad evenly among 4 plates. Top each salad with a grilled salmon fillet and sprinkle with the feta cheese. Serve immediately.

This Greek salad with grilled salmon is a great option for those with diabetes and high cholesterol for a few reasons:

- Salmon is an excellent source of heart•healthy omega•3 fatty acids.
- The fresh vegetables provide fiber, vitamins, minerals and antioxidants.
- The olive oil•based dressing is a healthier alternative to creamy dressings.
- The portion of 6 oz of salmon per serving provides a good amount of lean protein.
- The salad is low in carbs and high in fiber, making it diabetes•friendly.

92. Tuna and white bean salad with lemon vinaigrette

Ingredient:

- 1 (15 oz) can white beans, rinsed and drained
- 1 (5 oz) can tuna, drained and flaked
- 1/2 cup diced cucumber
- 1/4 cup diced red onion
- 2 tbsp chopped fresh parsley

Lemon Vinaigrette:
- 2 tbsp olive oil
- 1 tbsp lemon juice
- 1 tsp Dijon mustard
- 1 tsp honey
- 1/4 tsp salt
- 1/4 tsp black pepper

Instructions:

1. In a large bowl, combine the white beans, tuna, cucumber, red onion and parsley.

2. In a small bowl, whisk together the olive oil, lemon juice, Dijon, honey, salt and pepper to make the vinaigrette.

3. Pour the vinaigrette over the tuna and bean salad and toss gently to coat.

4. Serve the tuna and white bean salad chilled or at room temperature.

This tuna and white bean salad is a great option for those with diabetes and high cholesterol for a few reasons:

- Tuna is a lean protein that is low in saturated fat and cholesterol.
- White beans are a good source of fiber, protein and complex carbs, making them diabetes•friendly.
- The lemon vinaigrette is made with heart•healthy olive oil instead of mayonnaise or creamy dressings.
- The fresh vegetables and herbs provide antioxidants and nutrients.
- The portion size is balanced and appropriate for a main dish salad.

This salad is refreshing, flavorful and nutritious. Enjoy it as a light lunch or pair it with whole grain crackers for a satisfying and diabetes•friendly meal.

93. Roasted Brussels sprouts with pecans

Ingredient:

- 1 lb Brussels sprouts, trimmed and halved
- 2 tbsp olive oil
- 1/4 tsp salt
- 1/4 tsp black pepper
- 1/3 cup chopped pecans

Instructions:

1. Preheat oven to 400°F. Line a baking sheet with parchment paper.

2. In a large bowl, toss the Brussels sprouts with the olive oil, salt and pepper until evenly coated.

3. Spread the Brussels sprouts in a single layer on the prepared baking sheet.

4. Roast for 18•22 minutes, tossing halfway, until the Brussels sprouts are tender and lightly browned.

5. Remove the Brussels sprouts from the oven and sprinkle the chopped pecans over the top.

6. Return the pan to the oven and roast for an additional 3•5 minutes, until the pecans are lightly toasted.

7. Serve the roasted Brussels sprouts with pecans warm.

This roasted Brussels sprouts dish is a great option for those with diabetes and high cholesterol for a few reasons:

- Brussels sprouts are a low•carb, high•fiber vegetable that is diabetes•friendly.
- Pecans are a source of heart•healthy monounsaturated fats and antioxidants.
- Roasting the Brussels sprouts brings out their natural sweetness without the need for added sugars or sauces.
- The dish is naturally gluten•free and vegan.
- The portion size is balanced and appropriate for a diabetic•friendly side dish.

Enjoy these crispy, flavorful roasted Brussels sprouts with the added crunch of toasted pecans. They make a delicious and nutritious side dish to pair with lean proteins.

94. Baked salmon with teriyaki glaze

Ingredient:

- 4 (6 oz) salmon fillets
- 2 tbsp low•sodium soy sauce
- 1 tbsp rice vinegar
- 1 tbsp honey
- 1 tsp grated fresh ginger
- 1 clove garlic, minced
- 1/4 tsp red pepper flakes (optional)
- 1 tbsp sesame seeds (optional)

Instructions:

1. Preheat oven to 400°F. Line a baking sheet with parchment paper.

2. In a small bowl, whisk together the soy sauce, rice vinegar, honey, ginger, garlic and red pepper flakes (if using).

3. Place the salmon fillets on the prepared baking sheet. Brush the tops of the salmon with the teriyaki glaze.

4. Bake for 12•15 minutes, until the salmon is opaque and flakes easily with a fork.

5. Remove the baked salmon from the oven and sprinkle with the sesame seeds (if using). Serve the salmon warm, with any extra teriyaki glaze drizzled over the top.

This baked salmon with teriyaki glaze is a great option for those with diabetes and high cholesterol for a few reasons:

- Salmon is an excellent source of heart•healthy omega•3 fatty acids.
- The teriyaki glaze is made with low•sodium soy sauce, rice vinegar and a small amount of honey, rather than high•sugar store•bought teriyaki sauce.
- Baking the salmon is a healthier cooking method compared to frying.
- The portion size of 6 oz of salmon per serving provides a good amount of lean protein.
- The dish is low in carbs and high in healthy fats, making it diabetes•friendly.

Serve this flavorful baked salmon with a side of roasted vegetables or a fresh salad for a complete, diabetes•friendly and heart•healthy meal. Enjoy!

95. Shrimp and avocado salad with citrus dressing

Ingredient:

- 1 lb cooked shrimp, peeled and deveined
- 1 avocado, diced
- 1 cup cherry tomatoes, halved
- 1/2 cup diced cucumber
- 2 tbsp chopped fresh cilantro

Citrus Dressing:
- 2 tbsp olive oil
- 2 tbsp fresh orange juice
- 1 tbsp fresh lime juice
- 1 tsp Dijon mustard
- 1 tsp honey
- 1/4 tsp salt
- 1/4 tsp black pepper

Instructions:

1. In a large bowl, combine the cooked shrimp, avocado, tomatoes, cucumber and cilantro.

2. In a small bowl, whisk together all the dressing ingredients until well combined.

3. Pour the citrus dressing over the shrimp and avocado salad and toss gently to coat.

4. Serve the salad chilled or at room temperature.

This shrimp and avocado salad is a great option for those with diabetes and high cholesterol for a few reasons:

- Shrimp is a lean protein that is low in saturated fat and cholesterol.
- Avocado provides heart•healthy monounsaturated fats that can help lower cholesterol.
- The fresh vegetables and herbs provide fiber, vitamins, minerals and antioxidants.
- The citrus•based dressing is made with olive oil, which is a healthier fat compared to creamy dressings.
- The portion size is balanced and appropriate for a main dish salad.
- The dish is low in carbs and high in healthy fats, making it diabetes•friendly.

Enjoy this refreshing and nutritious shrimp and avocado salad as a light lunch or dinner. It's a great way to get in a variety of beneficial nutrients.

96. Eggplant rollatini with ricotta and spinach

Ingredient:

• 1 medium eggplant, sliced lengthwise into 1/4•inch thick slices
• 1 tbsp olive oil
• 1 cup part•skim ricotta cheese
• 1 cup chopped fresh spinach
• 1/4 cup grated Parmesan cheese
• 1 egg, lightly beaten
• 1 clove garlic, minced
• 1/4 tsp salt
• 1/4 tsp black pepper
• 1 cup marinara sauce

Instructions:

1. Preheat oven to 375°F. Lightly grease a baking dish.

2. Brush the eggplant slices lightly with olive oil on both sides. Place on a baking sheet and bake for 10•12 minutes, flipping halfway, until tender.

3. In a bowl, mix together the ricotta, spinach, Parmesan, egg, garlic, salt and pepper until well combined.

4. Spread 1/2 cup of the marinara sauce in the bottom of the prepared baking dish.

5. Place a heaping tablespoon of the ricotta•spinach mixture onto the end of each eggplant slice. Carefully roll up the eggplant and place seam•side down in the baking dish.

6. Top the eggplant rollatini with the remaining 1/2 cup of marinara sauce. Bake for 20•25 minutes, until heated through. Serve warm.

This eggplant rollatini dish is a great option for those with diabetes and high cholesterol for a few reasons:

• Eggplant is a low•carb, high•fiber vegetable that is diabetes•friendly.
• The use of part•skim ricotta and a small amount of Parmesan keeps the saturated fat and cholesterol content low.
• Spinach provides vitamins, minerals and antioxidants.
• Baking the eggplant instead of frying is a healthier cooking method.
• The marinara sauce provides lycopene and other beneficial plant compounds.
• The portion size is balanced and appropriate for a main dish.

97. Spinach and mushroom stuffed turkey breast

Ingredient:

- 1 lb boneless, skinless turkey breast
- 1 tbsp olive oil
- 8 oz sliced mushrooms
- 2 cups fresh spinach, chopped
- 2 cloves garlic, minced
- 1/4 cup low•fat ricotta cheese
- 2 tbsp grated Parmesan cheese
- 1 tsp dried thyme
- Salt and pepper to taste

Instructions:

1. Preheat oven to 375°F.

2. Slice the turkey breast horizontally to create a pocket, being careful not to cut all the way through.

3. In a skillet over medium heat, heat the olive oil. Add the mushrooms and sauté for 5•7 minutes, until softened.

4. Add the spinach and garlic to the skillet and cook for 2•3 minutes, until the spinach is wilted. Remove from heat and let cool slightly.

5. In a small bowl, mix together the sautéed spinach and mushroom mixture, ricotta cheese, Parmesan cheese, and thyme. Season with salt and pepper.

6. Stuff the spinach and mushroom mixture into the pocket of the turkey breast.

7. Place the stuffed turkey breast in a baking dish and bake for 30•35 minutes, until the internal temperature reaches 165°F.

8. Let the turkey rest for 5 minutes before slicing and serving.

This stuffed turkey breast is a great option for those with diabetes or high cholesterol, as it is high in protein, low in carbs, and contains healthy fats from the olive oil and ricotta cheese. The spinach and mushroom filling adds additional nutrients and fiber.

98. Chickpea and vegetable curry with coconut milk

Ingredient:

- 1 tbsp olive oil
- 1 onion, diced
- 3 cloves garlic, minced
- 1 tbsp grated fresh ginger
- 2 tsp curry powder
- 1 tsp ground cumin
- 1/2 tsp ground coriander
- 1/4 tsp cayenne pepper (optional, for spice)
- 1 can (15 oz) chickpeas, drained and rinsed
- 1 can (14 oz) diced tomatoes
- 1 can (13.5 oz) coconut milk
- 2 cups mixed vegetables (such as cauliflower, bell peppers, and spinach)
- Salt and pepper to taste
- Chopped fresh cilantro for garnish

Instructions:

1. In a large skillet or pot, heat the olive oil over medium heat. Add the onion and sauté for 5 minutes, until translucent.

2. Add the garlic and ginger and cook for 1 minute, until fragrant.

3. Stir in the curry powder, cumin, coriander, and cayenne (if using). Cook for 1 minute to toast the spices.

4. Add the chickpeas, diced tomatoes, and coconut milk. Bring to a simmer.

5. Add the mixed vegetables and cook for 10•15 minutes, until the vegetables are tender.

6. Season with salt and pepper to taste.

7. Serve the curry over cooked brown rice or quinoa, and garnish with chopped fresh cilantro.

This chickpea and vegetable curry is a great option for those with diabetes or high cholesterol, as it is high in fiber, protein, and healthy fats from the coconut milk, while being low in sodium and added sugars.

99. Turkey and quinoa stuffed bell peppers with salsa

Ingredient:

- 4 medium bell peppers, halved and seeded
- 1 lb ground turkey
- 1 cup cooked quinoa
- 1 cup diced tomatoes
- 1/2 cup diced onion
- 2 cloves garlic, minced
- 1 tsp chili powder
- 1 tsp cumin
- 1/4 cup chopped fresh cilantro
- Salt and pepper to taste
- 1 cup salsa (look for a low•sodium variety)

Instructions:

1. Preheat oven to 375°F.

2. In a large skillet over medium heat, cook the ground turkey until browned and cooked through, 5•7 minutes. Drain any excess fat.

3. Add the cooked quinoa, diced tomatoes, onion, garlic, chili powder, cumin, and cilantro to the skillet. Stir to combine and season with salt and pepper.

4. Stuff the turkey and quinoa mixture into the hollowed•out bell pepper halves.

5. Place the stuffed pepper halves in a baking dish and bake for 20•25 minutes, until the peppers are tender. Serve the stuffed peppers with the salsa on the side.

Nutritional Information (per serving):
Calories: 250
Total Fat: 8g
Saturated Fat: 2g
Cholesterol: 60mg

Sodium: 350mg
Carbohydrates: 25g
Fiber: 5g
Sugars: 7g
Protein: 22g

This dish is a great option for those with diabetes or high cholesterol, as it is high in protein, fiber, and healthy fats, while being low in sodium and added sugars. The salsa provides a flavorful and low•calorie topping.

100. Baked eggplant Parmesan with fresh basil

Ingredient:

- 2 medium eggplants, sliced into 1/2•inch thick rounds
- 1 tbsp olive oil
- 1 cup marinara sauce (look for a low•sodium variety)
- 1 cup shredded part•skim mozzarella cheese
- 1/4 cup grated Parmesan cheese
- 1/4 cup chopped fresh basil

Instructions:

1. Preheat oven to 375°F. Line a baking sheet with parchment paper.

2. Arrange the eggplant slices in a single layer on the prepared baking sheet. Brush the tops of the eggplant slices with the olive oil.

3. Bake the eggplant for 20•25 minutes, flipping halfway, until tender and lightly browned.

4. Remove the eggplant from the oven and top each slice with a spoonful of marinara sauce, followed by a sprinkle of mozzarella and Parmesan cheeses.

5. Return the eggplant to the oven and bake for an additional 10•15 minutes, until the cheese is melted and bubbly.

6. Remove the eggplant Parmesan from the oven and sprinkle with the chopped fresh basil. Serve immediately.

Nutritional Information (per serving):
Calories: 180
Total Fat: 9g
Saturated Fat: 3g

Cholesterol: 15mg
Sodium: 350mg
Carbohydrates: 15g
Fiber: 5g
Sugars: 7g
Protein: 10g

This baked eggplant Parmesan is a healthier alternative to the traditional fried version, as it is baked instead of fried and uses a lower•sodium marinara sauce. The fresh basil adds flavor without adding extra calories or sodium. This dish is a great option for those with diabetes or high cholesterol, as it is low in carbs, high in fiber, and contains healthy fats from the olive oil and cheese.

101. Grilled shrimp with pineapple salsa

Ingredient:

For the Shrimp:
- 1 lb large shrimp, peeled and deveined
- 1 tbsp olive oil
- 1 tsp chili powder
- 1/2 tsp garlic powder
- Salt and pepper to taste

For the Pineapple Salsa:
- 1 cup diced fresh pineapple
- 1/2 cup diced red onion
- 1/4 cup chopped fresh cilantro
- 1 jalapeño, seeded and finely chopped (optional, for spice)
- Juice of 1 lime
- Salt and pepper to taste

Instructions:

1. Make the pineapple salsa: In a medium bowl, combine the diced pineapple, red onion, cilantro, jalapeño (if using), and lime juice. Season with salt and pepper to taste. Cover and refrigerate until ready to serve.

2. Prepare the shrimp: In a large bowl, toss the shrimp with the olive oil, chili powder, garlic powder, salt, and pepper.

3. Preheat a grill or grill pan to medium•high heat.

4. Grill the shrimp for 2•3 minutes per side, or until they are opaque and cooked through.

5. Serve the grilled shrimp immediately, topped with the pineapple salsa.

Nutritional Information (per serving):
Calories: 200
Total Fat: 6g
Saturated Fat: 1g
Cholesterol: 170mg
Sodium: 350mg
Carbohydrates: 12g
Fiber: 2g
Sugars: 8g
Protein: 24g

This grilled shrimp with pineapple salsa is a great option for those with diabetes or high cholesterol. The shrimp provides a lean source of protein, while the pineapple salsa adds sweetness and fiber without too many additional calories or sodium. The dish is also low in saturated fat and high in healthy fats from the olive oil.

102. Cauliflower crust pizza with roasted vegetables

Ingredient:

For the Cauliflower Crust:
• 1 head of cauliflower, riced (about 3 cups riced cauliflower)
• 1 egg, beaten
• 1/2 cup shredded part•skim mozzarella cheese
• 2 tbsp grated Parmesan cheese
• 1 tsp dried oregano
• 1/2 tsp garlic powder
• Salt and pepper to taste

For the Toppings:
• 1 cup mixed roasted vegetables (such as bell peppers, zucchini, onions, and mushrooms)
• 1 cup marinara sauce (look for a low•sodium variety)
• 1 cup shredded part•skim mozzarella cheese
• 2 tbsp grated Parmesan cheese
• Fresh basil leaves for garnish

Instructions:
1. Preheat oven to 400°F. Line a baking sheet with parchment paper.

2. To make the cauliflower crust, place the riced cauliflower in a microwave•safe bowl and microwave for 5•7 minutes, until tender. Allow to cool slightly.

3. In a bowl, mix the cooked cauliflower, beaten egg, mozzarella, Parmesan, oregano, garlic powder, salt, and pepper until well combined.

4. Press the cauliflower mixture onto the prepared baking sheet, forming a thin, even crust.

5. Bake the crust for 20•25 minutes, until golden brown.

6. Top the baked crust with the marinara sauce, roasted vegetables, mozzarella, and Parmesan cheese. Bake the pizza for an additional 10•15 minutes, until the cheese is melted and bubbly. Remove the pizza from the oven and garnish with fresh basil leaves.

This cauliflower crust pizza is a great option for those with diabetes or high cholesterol, as it is low in carbs, high in fiber, and contains healthy fats from the cheese and vegetables. The roasted vegetables add additional nutrients and flavor without adding too many calories or sodium.

103. Greek yogurt with granola and berries

Ingredient:

- 1 cup plain, non•fat Greek yogurt
- 1/2 cup mixed berries (such as blueberries, raspberries, and/or strawberries)
- 1/4 cup low•sugar granola

Instructions:

1. In a parfait glass or bowl, layer the Greek yogurt, mixed berries, and granola.

2. Repeat the layers, ending with the granola on top. Serve immediately.

Nutritional Information (per serving):
Calories: 200
Total Fat: 2g
Saturated Fat: 0g
Cholesterol: 10mg
Sodium: 80mg
Carbohydrates: 28g
Fiber: 5g
Sugars: 15g
Protein: 18g

This Greek yogurt parfait is an excellent choice for those with diabetes or high cholesterol for several reasons:

1. Greek yogurt is high in protein and low in carbs, making it a great option for those with diabetes. The protein helps to keep blood sugar levels stable.

2. The berries provide fiber, vitamins, and antioxidants without adding too many carbs or calories.

3. The low•sugar granola adds a crunchy texture and a touch of sweetness, without spiking blood sugar levels.

4. The overall dish is low in saturated fat, sodium, and added sugars, which is important for those with high cholesterol.

This parfait can be enjoyed as a healthy breakfast, snack, or dessert. It's a simple, yet delicious way to incorporate nutrient•dense ingredients into your diet.

104. Baked chicken with rosemary and garlic

Ingredient:

- 4 boneless, skinless chicken breasts
- 2 tbsp olive oil
- 3 cloves garlic, minced
- 2 tsp dried rosemary
- 1 tsp paprika
- Salt and pepper to taste

Instructions:

1. Preheat your oven to 400°F. Line a baking sheet with parchment paper or a silicone baking mat.

2. In a small bowl, combine the olive oil, minced garlic, dried rosemary, paprika, salt, and pepper.

3. Place the chicken breasts on the prepared baking sheet and brush or rub the garlic•rosemary mixture all over the chicken.

4. Bake the chicken for 25•30 minutes, or until it reaches an internal temperature of 165°F. Remove the chicken from the oven and let it rest for 5 minutes before serving.

This baked chicken dish is an excellent choice for those with diabetes or high cholesterol for several reasons:

1. Chicken is a lean protein that is low in carbs and high in protein, making it a great option for those with diabetes.

2. The use of olive oil provides healthy monounsaturated fats, which can help lower cholesterol levels.

3. The dish is low in sodium, with only 150mg per serving, which is important for those with high blood pressure or heart disease.

4. The herbs and spices, such as rosemary and paprika, add flavor without the need for additional salt or unhealthy seasonings.

Serve this baked chicken with a side of roasted vegetables or a fresh salad for a complete and nutritious meal.

105. Lentil and vegetable stew with turmeric

Ingredient:

- 1 cup dry brown or green lentils, rinsed
- 4 cups low•sodium vegetable broth
- 1 tbsp olive oil
- 1 onion, diced
- 3 cloves garlic, minced
- 2 carrots, peeled and diced
- 2 celery stalks, diced
- 1 cup diced butternut squash
- 1 tsp ground turmeric
- 1 tsp ground cumin
- 1/2 tsp ground coriander
- 1/4 tsp cayenne pepper (optional)
- 1/4 tsp salt
- 1/4 tsp black pepper
- 2 cups chopped kale or spinach
- 2 tbsp chopped fresh cilantro

Instructions:

1. In a large pot, combine the lentils and vegetable broth. Bring to a boil, then reduce heat and simmer for 15•20 minutes, until lentils are tender.

2. In a separate large pot or Dutch oven, heat the olive oil over medium heat. Add the onion and sauté for 3•4 minutes until translucent.

3. Add the garlic, carrots, celery and butternut squash. Cook for 5•7 minutes, stirring occasionally, until the vegetables start to soften.

4. Stir in the turmeric, cumin, coriander, cayenne (if using), salt and pepper. Cook for 1 minute to toast the spices.

5. Add the cooked lentils and their broth to the vegetable mixture. Bring to a simmer and cook for 10•15 minutes, until the vegetables are tender.

6. Stir in the chopped kale or spinach and cook for 2•3 minutes until wilted. Remove from heat and stir in the fresh cilantro. Serve the lentil and vegetable stew warm.

106. Turkey and vegetable stir•fry with quinoa

Ingredient:

- 1 cup uncooked quinoa
- 1 lb ground turkey
- 2 tbsp low•sodium soy sauce
- 1 tbsp rice vinegar
- 1 tsp sesame oil
- 1 tsp grated fresh ginger
- 2 cloves garlic, minced
- 2 cups mixed vegetables (such as broccoli, bell peppers, and snow peas)
- 2 green onions, sliced
- Salt and pepper to taste

Instructions:

1. Cook the quinoa according to package instructions. Set aside.

2. In a large skillet or wok, cook the ground turkey over medium•high heat, breaking it up with a wooden spoon, until browned and cooked through, about 5•7 minutes.

3. In a small bowl, whisk together the soy sauce, rice vinegar, sesame oil, ginger, and garlic.

4. Add the mixed vegetables to the skillet with the cooked turkey. Pour the soy sauce mixture over the top and stir to combine.

5. Cook the stir•fry for 5•7 minutes, or until the vegetables are tender•crisp. Serve the turkey and vegetable stir•fry over the cooked quinoa, garnished with the sliced green onions.

This turkey and vegetable stir•fry with quinoa is an excellent choice for those with diabetes or high cholesterol for several reasons:

1. Ground turkey is a lean protein that is low in fat and high in protein, making it a great option for those with diabetes.
2. The quinoa provides a source of complex carbohydrates, fiber, and protein, which can help regulate blood sugar levels.
3. The stir•fried vegetables add fiber, vitamins, and minerals without too many additional calories or carbs.
4. The dish is low in sodium, with only 400mg per serving, which is important for those with high blood pressure or heart disease.

107. Baked trout with pistachio crust

Ingredient:

- 4 trout fillets (about 1 lb total)
- 1/2 cup shelled, unsalted pistachios, finely chopped
- 2 tbsp whole wheat breadcrumbs
- 1 tbsp grated lemon zest
- 1 tbsp chopped fresh parsley
- 1 tbsp olive oil
- Salt and pepper to taste

Instructions:

1. Preheat your oven to 400°F. Line a baking sheet with parchment paper.

2. In a small bowl, mix together the chopped pistachios, breadcrumbs, lemon zest, parsley, and olive oil. Season with salt and pepper.

3. Place the trout fillets on the prepared baking sheet. Evenly distribute the pistachio mixture on top of the trout, pressing it gently to adhere.

4. Bake the trout for 12•15 minutes, or until the fish flakes easily with a fork and the crust is golden brown. Serve the baked trout immediately.

This baked trout with a pistachio crust is an excellent choice for those with diabetes or high cholesterol for several reasons:

1. Trout is a lean, oily fish that is high in heart•healthy omega•3 fatty acids, which can help lower triglyceride and cholesterol levels.

2. The pistachio crust provides a crunchy texture and healthy fats, without adding too many carbs or calories.

3. The dish is low in sodium, with only 200mg per serving, which is important for those with high blood pressure or heart disease.

4. The lemon zest and parsley add flavor without the need for additional salt or unhealthy seasonings.

Serve this baked trout with a side of roasted vegetables or a fresh salad for a complete and nutritious meal.

108. Spinach and feta stuffed chicken thighs

Ingredient:

- 6 boneless, skinless chicken thighs
- 1 cup fresh spinach, chopped
- 1/2 cup crumbled feta cheese
- 2 cloves garlic, minced
- 1 tbsp olive oil
- 1 tsp dried oregano
- Salt and pepper to taste

Instructions:

1. Preheat your oven to 400°F. Line a baking sheet with parchment paper.

2. In a small bowl, mix together the chopped spinach, crumbled feta, minced garlic, 1 tsp of the olive oil, and the dried oregano. Season with salt and pepper.

3. Carefully slice each chicken thigh horizontally, creating a pocket. Stuff each thigh with the spinach and feta mixture, pressing it in gently.

4. Place the stuffed chicken thighs on the prepared baking sheet. Drizzle the remaining 2 tsp of olive oil over the top of the chicken.

5. Bake the chicken for 25•30 minutes, or until the chicken is cooked through and the internal temperature reaches 165°F.

6. Remove the chicken from the oven and let it rest for 5 minutes before serving.

This spinach and feta stuffed chicken thighs dish is an excellent choice for those with diabetes or high cholesterol for several reasons:

1. Chicken thighs are a lean protein that is low in carbs, making them a great option for those with diabetes.
2. The spinach and feta filling provides a source of healthy fats, fiber, and vitamins without adding too many additional carbs or calories.
3. The dish is relatively low in sodium, with only 350mg per serving, which is important for those with high blood pressure or heart disease.
4. The use of olive oil instead of butter or other unhealthy fats helps to keep the dish heart•healthy.

Serve this stuffed chicken with a side of roasted vegetables or a fresh salad for a complete and nutritious meal.

109. Quinoa and black bean salad with lime dressing

Ingredient:

- 1 cup uncooked quinoa, rinsed
- 1 (15 oz) can black beans, drained and rinsed
- 1 cup diced cucumber
- 1 cup diced tomatoes
- 1/2 cup diced red onion
- 1/4 cup chopped fresh cilantro
- 2 tbsp olive oil
- 2 tbsp lime juice
- 1 tsp honey
- 1/2 tsp ground cumin
- Salt and pepper to taste

Instructions:

1. Cook the quinoa according to package instructions. Allow to cool.

2. In a large bowl, combine the cooked quinoa, black beans, cucumber, tomatoes, red onion, and cilantro.

3. In a small bowl, whisk together the olive oil, lime juice, honey, and cumin. Season with salt and pepper.

4. Pour the dressing over the quinoa and bean mixture and toss gently to coat. Refrigerate the salad for at least 30 minutes to allow the flavors to meld. Serve chilled or at room temperature.

This quinoa and black bean salad is an excellent choice for those with diabetes or high cholesterol for several reasons:

1. Quinoa is a whole grain that is high in fiber and protein, which can help regulate blood sugar levels.
2. Black beans are a great source of plant•based protein and fiber, which can also help manage blood sugar and cholesterol levels.
3. The vegetables, such as cucumber, tomatoes, and onion, provide additional fiber, vitamins, and minerals without adding too many carbs or calories.
4. The lime dressing is made with healthy fats from olive oil and a touch of honey for sweetness, without the need for added sugars or sodium.

This salad can be enjoyed as a main dish or a side, and it's a great option for meal prepping or bringing to potlucks and gatherings.

110. Turkey and avocado salad with cilantro lime dressing

Ingredient:

- 2 cups cooked turkey breast, diced
- 1 avocado, diced
- 1 cup cherry tomatoes, halved
- 1/2 cup diced cucumber
- 1/4 cup diced red onion
- 2 tbsp chopped fresh cilantro
- Juice of 1 lime
- 1 tbsp olive oil
- 1 tsp Dijon mustard
- 1 tsp honey
- Salt and pepper to taste

Instructions:

1. In a large bowl, combine the diced turkey, avocado, cherry tomatoes, cucumber, and red onion.

2. In a small bowl, whisk together the lime juice, olive oil, Dijon mustard, and honey. Season with salt and pepper.

3. Pour the dressing over the salad and toss gently to coat. Sprinkle the chopped cilantro over the top. Serve immediately.

Nutritional Information (per serving):
Calories: 220
Total Fat: 12g
Saturated Fat: 2g
Cholesterol: 45mg
Sodium: 220mg
Carbohydrates: 10g
Fiber: 5g
Sugars: 4g
Protein: 20g

This salad is a great option for those with diabetes or high cholesterol, as it is high in protein, healthy fats from the avocado, and low in carbs and sodium. The cilantro lime dressing adds flavor without adding too many additional calories or unhealthy ingredients.

111. Baked tilapia with mango salsa

Ingredient:

For the Tilapia:
- 4 tilapia fillets (about 1 lb total)
- 1 tbsp olive oil
- 1 tsp chili powder
- 1/2 tsp garlic powder
- Salt and pepper to taste

For the Mango Salsa:
- 1 ripe mango, diced
- 1/2 red onion, diced
- 1 jalapeño, seeded and finely chopped (optional, for spice)
- 1/4 cup chopped fresh cilantro
- 2 tbsp lime juice
- Salt and pepper to taste

Instructions:

1. Preheat your oven to 400°F. Line a baking sheet with parchment paper.

2. Make the mango salsa: In a medium bowl, combine the diced mango, red onion, jalapeño (if using), cilantro, and lime juice. Season with salt and pepper to taste. Cover and refrigerate until ready to serve.

3. Prepare the tilapia: Place the tilapia fillets on the prepared baking sheet. Brush the fillets with the olive oil and sprinkle with the chili powder, garlic powder, salt, and pepper.

4. Bake the tilapia for 12•15 minutes, or until it flakes easily with a fork and reaches an internal temperature of 145°F. Serve the baked tilapia immediately, topped with the mango salsa.

This baked tilapia with mango salsa is an excellent choice for those with diabetes or high cholesterol for several reasons:
1. Tilapia is a lean, mild•flavored fish that is low in calories and high in protein, making it a great option for those with diabetes.

2. The mango salsa provides a sweet and tangy flavor without the need for added sugars or unhealthy sauces.

3. The dish is relatively low in sodium, with only 200mg per serving, which is important for those with high blood pressure or heart disease.

4. The use of olive oil and the lack of heavy creams or butter keeps the dish heart•healthy.

Serve this baked tilapia with mango salsa alongside a side of roasted vegetables or a fresh salad for a complete and nutritious meal.

112. Grilled chicken with peach chutney

Ingredient:

For the Peach Chutney:
- 2 ripe peaches, diced
- 1/2 red onion, diced
- 2 tbsp apple cider vinegar
- 1 tbsp honey
- 1 tsp grated fresh ginger
- 1/4 tsp ground cumin
- Salt and pepper to taste

For the Chicken:
- 4 boneless, skinless chicken breasts
- 1 tbsp olive oil
- Salt and pepper to taste

Instructions:

1. Make the peach chutney: In a small saucepan, combine the diced peaches, red onion, apple cider vinegar, honey, ginger, and cumin. Bring the mixture to a simmer over medium heat, then reduce the heat and let it cook for 10•15 minutes, stirring occasionally, until the chutney has thickened. Season with salt and pepper to taste. Set aside.

2. Prepare the chicken: Preheat your grill or grill pan to medium•high heat.

3. Brush the chicken breasts with the olive oil and season with salt and pepper.

4. Grill the chicken for 5•7 minutes per side, or until it reaches an internal temperature of 165°F. Serve the grilled chicken topped with the peach chutney.

This grilled chicken with peach chutney is an excellent choice for those with diabetes or high cholesterol for several reasons:

1. Chicken is a lean protein that is low in carbs, making it a great option for those with diabetes.

2. The peach chutney provides a sweet and tangy flavor without the need for added sugars or unhealthy sauces.

3. The dish is relatively low in sodium, with only 200mg per serving, which is important for those with high blood pressure or heart disease.

4. The use of olive oil and the lack of heavy creams or butter keeps the dish heart•healthy.

Serve this grilled chicken with a side of roasted vegetables or a fresh salad for a complete and nutritious meal.

113. Tofu and vegetable stir-fry with ginger soy sauce

Ingredient:

- 1 block (14 oz) extra•firm tofu, cubed
- 2 tbsp sesame oil, divided
- 2 cups mixed vegetables (such as broccoli, bell peppers, and snow peas), chopped
- 2 cloves garlic, minced
- 1 tbsp grated fresh ginger
- 2 tbsp low•sodium soy sauce
- 1 tbsp rice vinegar
- 1 tsp honey
- Salt and pepper to taste
- Chopped green onions for garnish (optional)

Instructions:

1. In a large skillet or wok, heat 1 tbsp of the sesame oil over medium•high heat. Add the cubed tofu and cook, stirring occasionally, until lightly browned on all sides, about 5•7 minutes. Transfer the tofu to a plate and set aside.

2. In the same skillet, heat the remaining 1 tbsp of sesame oil. Add the chopped vegetables and sauté for 3•5 minutes, until they are tender•crisp.

3. Add the minced garlic and grated ginger to the skillet and cook for 1 minute, until fragrant.

4. In a small bowl, whisk together the soy sauce, rice vinegar, and honey.

5. Add the cooked tofu back to the skillet and pour the soy sauce mixture over the top. Toss everything together and cook for an additional 2•3 minutes, until the sauce has thickened slightly.

6. Season the stir•fry with salt and pepper to taste. Serve the tofu and vegetable stir•fry hot, garnished with chopped green onions if desired.

This tofu and vegetable stir•fry with a ginger soy sauce is an excellent choice for those with diabetes or high cholesterol for several reasons:

1. Tofu is a plant•based protein that is low in carbs and high in fiber, making it a great option for those with diabetes.
2. The vegetables provide additional fiber, vitamins, and minerals without adding too many carbs or calories.

114. Zucchini noodles with creamy Alfredo sauce

Ingredient:

- 3 medium zucchini, spiralized or julienned into noodles
- 1 tbsp olive oil
- 2 cloves garlic, minced
- 1/2 cup low•fat milk
- 2 oz low•fat cream cheese, softened
- 1/4 cup grated Parmesan cheese
- 2 tbsp chopped fresh parsley
- Salt and pepper to taste

Instructions:

1. In a large skillet, heat the olive oil over medium heat. Add the zucchini noodles and sauté for 3•5 minutes, until tender but still slightly crunchy. Transfer the zucchini noodles to a plate and set aside.

2. In the same skillet, add the minced garlic and cook for 1 minute, until fragrant.

3. Whisk in the low•fat milk and cream cheese. Cook, stirring frequently, until the cream cheese has melted and the sauce is smooth, about 2•3 minutes.

4. Remove the skillet from the heat and stir in the grated Parmesan cheese. Season with salt and pepper to taste.

5. Add the sautéed zucchini noodles back to the skillet and toss to coat with the Alfredo sauce. Serve the zucchini noodles with Alfredo sauce immediately, garnished with chopped fresh parsley.

This zucchini noodle dish with a creamy Alfredo sauce is an excellent choice for those with diabetes or high cholesterol for several reasons:

1. Zucchini noodles are a low•carb, high•fiber alternative to traditional pasta, making them a great option for those with diabetes.
2. The Alfredo sauce is made with low•fat milk and cream cheese, reducing the amount of saturated fat and calories compared to a traditional Alfredo sauce.
3. The dish is relatively low in sodium, with only 300mg per serving, which is important for those with high blood pressure or heart disease.
4. The addition of fresh parsley provides antioxidants and additional flavor without the need for excessive salt or unhealthy seasonings.

115. Cauliflower rice with spicy roasted chickpeas

Ingredient:

For the Chickpeas:
- 1 (15 oz) can chickpeas, drained and rinsed
- 1 tbsp olive oil
- 1 tsp chili powder
- 1/2 tsp paprika
- 1/4 tsp cayenne pepper (optional, for extra spice)
- Salt and pepper to taste

For the Cauliflower Rice:
- 1 head of cauliflower, riced
(about 4 cups riced cauliflower)
- 1 tbsp olive oil
- 2 cloves garlic, minced
- 1/2 cup diced onion
- 1/4 cup chopped fresh parsley
- Salt and pepper to taste

Instructions:

1. Preheat your oven to 400°F. Line a baking sheet with parchment paper.

2. In a bowl, toss the drained and rinsed chickpeas with the olive oil, chili powder, paprika, cayenne (if using), salt, and pepper. Spread the chickpeas in a single layer on the prepared baking sheet.

3. Roast the chickpeas for 20•25 minutes, stirring halfway, until crispy.

4. While the chickpeas are roasting, prepare the cauliflower rice. In a large skillet, heat the olive oil over medium heat. Add the minced garlic and diced onion, and sauté for 2•3 minutes, until fragrant and translucent.

5. Add the riced cauliflower to the skillet and cook for 5•7 minutes, stirring occasionally, until the cauliflower is tender.

6. Remove the skillet from the heat and stir in the chopped fresh parsley. Season with salt and pepper to taste. Serve the cauliflower rice topped with the spicy roasted chickpeas.

This cauliflower rice with spicy roasted chickpeas is an excellent choice for those with diabetes or high cholesterol for several reasons:

1. Cauliflower rice is a low•carb, high•fiber alternative to traditional rice, making it a great option for those with diabetes.
2. Chickpeas are a good source of plant•based protein and fiber, which can help regulate blood sugar levels and support heart health.
3. The dish is relatively low in sodium, with only 350mg per serving, which is important for those with high blood pressure or heart disease.
4. The use of olive oil and spices adds flavor without the need for excessive salt or unhealthy fats.

As we conclude the **"Cookbook For Diabetics and High Cholesterol: 115+ Wholesome Recipes for Diabetics and Lowering Cholesterol,"** *we hope you've found inspiration and practical guidance in creating delicious meals that support your health goals. Managing diabetes and high cholesterol requires thoughtful choices, especially when it comes to what we eat, and this cookbook has been crafted to make those choices easier and more enjoyable.*

Throughout these pages, you've discovered over 115 recipes that emphasize wholesome ingredients, balanced nutrition, and culinary creativity. From nourishing breakfasts to satisfying dinners and tempting desserts, each recipe has been designed not only to delight your taste buds but also to contribute positively to your overall well-being.

Beyond the recipes, we've aimed to equip you with knowledge and tips to navigate your dietary journey with confidence. Whether you're new to managing these conditions or seeking fresh ideas to expand your culinary repertoire, our hope is that this book has been a trusted companion in your kitchen.

Remember, cooking for health doesn't have to be bland or restrictive. With the right ingredients and techniques, you can savor flavorful meals that also support your diabetes management and cholesterol-lowering efforts. Embrace the joy of cooking and the satisfaction of nourishing yourself and your loved ones with meals that promote wellness.

Thank you for embarking on this culinary adventure with us. Here's to continued good health, delicious meals, and the power of wholesome cooking.

Happy cooking!